MEDITERRANEAN DIET COOKBOOK FOR BEGINNERS:

150 OF THE GREATEST AND MOST LOVED MEDITERRANEAN DIET RECIPES SELECTED FOR YOU. EASY, HEALTHY RECIPES TO LOSE WEIGHT, WITH NEW IDEAS AND TIPS YOU'LL LOVE.

BEATRICE MORELLI

Table Of Contents

Introduction

Thank you for choosing this guide. I have more for you on the Mediterranean diet, kindly refer to my other book in which the Mediterranean diet is widely discussed, *Mediterranean Diet for Beginners: Why Mediterranean Cooking Is the Healthiest Method to Lose Weight. Your Complete 21-Day Diet Meal Plan to Make You Fall in Love with a Unique Dining Experience.*

The Mediterranean diet is primarily a heart-healthy eating plan based on the traditional food, drinks, meals, and recipes of the countries surrounding the Mediterranean Sea. To put it simply, the Mediterranean diet is adopting the Mediterranean cuisine and cooking style.

The Mediterranean diet is not a diet per se. You don't really go on a diet. Rather, the "diet" is a lifestyle that has been studied and noted to be as one of the healthiest in the world.

This eating plan or model does not only include healthy food, but it also involves physical activities, eating meals with family and friends, and drinking wine in moderation.

Just as important as eating healthy, the Mediterranean diet also emphasizes on preparing flavorful, delicious meals and dishes. If you are a novice in "eating like a Greek" you may think that the Mediterranean cooking-style is complex, but the beautiful fact about this diet, once you have begun the lifestyle changes and adopted the Mediterranean eating habit, this eating plan is very simple and fun. You'll find that there are tons of easy Mediterranean dishes and it does not take much to improve your health and lose weight and enjoy fabulous dishes right in the comforts of your own home.

One common thing which connects them all is the food they consume and the way it is consumed. Legumes, vegetable, nuts, fish, grains, cereals, fruits, beans, and good Fats, these are things which mainly forms the Mediterranean diet. So, it guarantees a good amount of Fibers along with all the macronutrients like carbohydrates, Proteins, Fat, etc.

Several scientific studies have proven that the Mediterranean diet does provide all the essential nutrients which can help the body against genetic complexities, early signs of aging, gut ailments, mental illness, skin problems, and other diseases. A group of experts from America studied this diet with respect to its Fat content and its possible health impacts. And the results showed that the diet was effective in preventing cardiovascular diseases and increased the average age of life expectancies in the areas under study.

Since the major focus of the Mediterranean diet is on plant-based products, like grains, seeds, fruits, vegetables, oils, this is probably the true reason that it is full of important nutrients and devoid of Fats or bad cholesterol and harmful toxins. From vegetables to grains and fruits, to dairy to meat and seafood, we can experience all using this diet, but it must be in a perfectly balanced proportion.

Health Benefits And Why It Works

The tradition and history of the Mediterranean diet come from the traditional food and social patterns of the regions of southern Italy, Greece, Turkey, and Spain. This is why the Mediterranean diet is not even a "diet", but rather a lifestyle. For thousands of years, the inhabitants of the Mediterranean coast have eaten a diet rich in Fiber-diet of fruits and vegetables, Proteins and Fats in moderation, and a glass of locally made wine on occasion to complete a meal.

The Mediterranean diet has several advantages. Ingredients are now available and delicious dishes can be prepared quickly and easily. Here are some of the most important benefits of the Mediterranean diet:

- Low in processed foods and sugar

The diet consists of natural foods, including olive oil, legumes such as peas and beans, fruits and vegetables, unrefined grain products and small portions of animal products (always organic and locally produced). For something sweet, the Mediterranean people love fruit or small portions of homemade desserts with natural sweeteners such as honey.

In addition to plant foods, moderate consumption of locally caught fish and cow, goat, or sheep cheese and yogurt are other important components of the diet. Fish such as sardines and anchovies are a central part of the diet, which generally contains less meat than many Western diets.

Although most Mediterranean people are not vegetarians, the diet favors only low consumption of meat and heavier meals, opting for lighter and healthier fish options. This can be beneficial for people who want to lose weight and improve heart health, cholesterol and omega-3 Fatty acid intake.

- Assists healthy weight loss

If you want to lose weight without being hungry and maintain it in a realistic way throughout your life, this may be the answer. The diet is durable and valuable. It has been successfully used by many people around the world, especially because it helps to control weight and reduce Fat consumption naturally and simply through the consumption of nutrient-rich foods.

The Mediterranean diet can be interpreted differently, whether you prefer to eat fewer carbohydrates, less Protein, or somewhere in between. The diet focuses on the consumption of healthy Fats, while carbohydrates are kept relatively low, and the consumption of foods high in high-quality Protein is improved. If you prefer Protein to legumes and cereals, you can lose weight in a healthy, non-deprived way, with a large amount of high-quality seafood and dairy products (which at the same time offer other benefits such as omega-3s and often probiotics).

Fish, dairy products and meat contain the healthy Fatty acids that the body needs. They work to help you feel full, control your weight gain, regulate your blood sugar, your mood, and your energy level. But if you are more of a plant-based consumer, legumes and whole grains (especially if they are soaked and sprouted) are also good options.

- Improves heart health

Research shows that greater compliance with the traditional Mediterranean diet, which includes monounsaturated and omega-3 Fatty acids, is associated with a significant reduction in mortality, especially heart disease.

Olive oil is also beneficial for reducing hypertension because nitric oxide is more bioavailable, allowing it to dilate blood vessels and keep it clean. Another element of protection is that it helps to combat the effects of oxidation that promotes disease and improves endothelial function. People in the Mediterranean generally have no difficulty maintaining healthy cholesterol levels because they eat lots of healthy

Fats.

● Helps fight cancer

A plant-based diet rich in fruits and vegetables is the cornerstone of the Mediterranean diet. It can help fight cancer, as it provides antioxidants, protects DNA from damage, stops cell mutation, reduces inflammation and slows tumor growth. Many studies indicate that olive oil can also be a natural treatment for cancer and can reduce the risk of colon cancer. It could have a protective effect on the development of cancer cells because it reduces inflammation and oxidative stress, while promoting a glycemic balance and healthy weight.

● Prevents or treats diabetes

The Mediterranean diet is anti-inflammatory and may help fight diseases related to chronic inflammation, including metabolic syndrome and type 2 diabetes. It regulates excess insulin, a hormone that regulates the blood sugar level.

The Mediterranean diet is low in sugar because the only sugar present comes mainly from fruits, wine, and sometimes local desserts. In terms of drinks, many people also drink lots of fresh water, coffee and red wine. Sodas and sugary drinks are not as popular in the Mediterranean as they are in the United States.

Although some Mediterranean diets contain a large number of carbohydrates, such as pasta and bread, being active and consuming minimal amounts of sugar means that insulin resistance is rare in these countries. The Mediterranean eating style helps to prevent peaks and troughs in the blood sugar level, which reduces energy and affects your mood. All of these different factors contribute to the diabetes prevention benefits of this diet.

● Protects cognitive health and improves mood

Eating a Mediterranean diet can be a natural treatment for Parkinson's disease, a great way to protect your memory and a step in the right direction to treat Alzheimer's disease and dementia naturally. Cognitive impairment can occur when the brain does not receive enough dopamine, a chemical substance that is essential for the body to function properly.

It is known that healthy Fats such as olive oil and nuts, as well as many anti-inflammatory fruits and vegetables, fight age-related cognitive impairment. This helps to counteract the harmful effects of exposure to toxicity, free radicals and poor diets that cause inflammation or food allergies, which can contribute to the deterioration of brain function. This is one of the reasons why respect for the Mediterranean diet is linked to lower rates for Alzheimer's disease.

Probiotic foods such as yogurt and kefir also help to develop a healthy digestive system, which we now know are related to cognitive functions, memory and mood.

- Increases longevity

A diet rich in fresh plant-based foods and healthy Fats is a winning combination for long life. Monounsaturated
Fatty acids, found in olive oil and some nuts, are the main source of Fat in the Mediterranean diet. Time and time again, studies have shown that monounsaturated Fats are associated with low levels of heart disease, cancer, depression, cognitive diseases, Alzheimer's, inflammatory diseases, etc. Currently, heart disease is by far the leading cause of death in developed countries.

- Relieves stress and promotes relaxation

Another important factor is that this diet encourages people to spend time in nature, to sleep well, and to work together to create healthy home cooked meals. All are great ways to relieve stress and, as a result, to prevent inflammation. In general, people living in these areas eat food surrounded by family and friends (rather than alone or on the road) and spend time laughing, dancing, gardening and enjoying life.

Chronic stress can affect your quality of life, your weight and your health. People who eat at a slow pace, consume natural, local foods and engage in regular physical activity are more likely to maintain a good mood.

The Mediterranean diet includes love and fascination for wine, especially red wine, which is considered moderately beneficial and protective. For example, red wine can help fight obesity.

- Helps fight depression

According to a study, those who follow the Mediterranean diet can help reduce the risk of depression. Researchers participating in the study examined the mental health effects of adherence to various diets, such as the Mediterranean diet, the Healthy Eating Index (HEI) diet, Dietary approaches to stop hypertension (DASH diet), and the rate of inflammation of the diet. They found that the risk of depression decreased further when people followed a traditional Mediterranean diet and generally ate various anti-inflammatory foods.

Mediterranean Diet Basics

Raw Plant Foods

As a basis of Mediterranean Diet, it's highly recommended a green leaf before each meal. Raw plant foods mean in their interpretation of "live" food, which in nature contains all the vital substances for the body. In addition, raw food is given even greater importance in the prevention of health and the treatment of disease. Due to the content of ballast substances, raw food stimulates regular stools, while refined and denatured food is often the cause of constipation—a widespread and far from harmless affliction today.

An extremely important property of raw food is its beneficial effect on metabolic processes. Raw food increases the speed of their flow and stimulates a thorough cleaning of the body from toxins and poisons, thereby increasing its defenses. Introduction to the diet of raw plant food in sufficient volume is of great importance for the heart and blood vessels, since such food normalizes the level of Fat in the blood and largely counteracts the tendency to clotting blood that appears after traditional meals. This makes the daily intake of raw plant foods before each meal indispensable in the prevention of health. In general, raw food should be in the daily diet 30-50%.

To provide yourself with all the nutrients and vitally necessary substances, use the whole variety of plant products. They must harmoniously complement each other. Use them as fresh as possible (right from the garden! right from the branch of the tree!). Love their natural taste. Therefore, to avoid nutrient deficiencies, every day you should have fresh fruits, vegetables, root vegetables, greens, and salads on your table. True, raw plant foods cannot serve as the only source of nutrition for a long period since they are not able to provide the body with everything necessary. Only if necessary, the doctor may prescribe as a therapeutic agent a diet consisting exclusively of raw plant foods for a long time.

Cereal Products

Use whole grains for cooking cereal dishes. Today's white flour products polished rice, any refined cereal products contain only traces of vital substances and therefore donate so-called empty calories to the body—the reason for being overweight.

If you cannot find such products for sale or they are very expensive, then I suggest purchasing a special small mill for the coarse grinding of grain. Such a "semi-natural farm" will definitely be more economically advantageous than the purchase of similar products in super and hypermarkets or in specialized health food stores.

True, in the consumption of grain should—as in everything else—abide by the measure. They acidify the body, their frequent consumption of canned food, under certain circumstances, increase susceptibility to disease.

Milk and Lactic Products

They are indispensable for covering the body's need for Proteins. Therefore, they must be introduced into the diet in sufficient quantities, even with vegan food. Adults, however, it is recommended to consume daily no more than 1/4 liter of milk, and it is better unpasteurized, not denatured due to heating, especially not sterilized. The greater effect gives an introduction to the menu of fermented milk products such as cottage cheese, whey, buttermilk, yogurt, fermented milk, kefir and other similar. For example, they can be used to prepare delicious salads, fruit and grain dishes.

Melted and hard cheeses in healthy nutrition are used sparingly, as they usually contain a lot of Fat and salt.

Eggs

Eggs are an indispensable high-grade food, but it is recommended to eat no more than 1-2 pieces per week. Daily consumption of eggs is discouraged due to cholesterol content, contributing primarily to calcification of the arteries. Eggs are also recommended to be taken "from under the hen", that is, carried from birds, which are kept in natural conditions, and not in poultry farms. Poultry products do not meet the requirements for healthy nutrition.

Meat and Fish

Meat, fish, and sausages are the usual food of Americans—the main part of it. However, frequent consumption of products of this group contributes to the emergence of widespread diseases of civilization. In a Mediterranean diet full meal these foods are highly limited. If it is difficult for you to completely abandon them, then include preferably fish and seafood instead red meat no more than 2 times a week in the menu, and then in moderate quantities as an appendix to vegetable food, and not the main dish.

If you can't replace totally red meat it is desirable to buy meat from animals grown in natural conditions, kept on a natural, vegetable diet without useless (if not to say harmful!) feed additives, without drugs. At first glance, it seems that this is a pipe dream, but in provincial American cities, such a service is not uncommon: local farmers feed calves, pigs, poultry to order, and you can check the quality of Fattening at any time, arriving in the village by bus or car. As a rule, you can buy fresh milk and eggs from local farmers.

Winter Delicacies

Now, almost at any time of the year, you can buy plant food, but in winter, it is more expensive, so you can replenish the diet with dried or frozen vegetables, fruits, berries, greens, and canned food from them.

However, products of quick freezing should be preferred, since the loss of vital substances during freezing occurs very slowly, whereas at the first stage of canning, which is associated with heating and boiling, much more vital substances are destroyed. Since the amount of losses in canned food almost stabilizes, and in products of fast freezing losses continue—slowly but constantly, then during storage for a long period, canned food can easily compete with products of fast freezing. However, neither one nor the other will ever be able to completely replace raw plant foods.

But correctly dried and stored in optimal conditions, fruits, vegetables, herbs for seasoning retain vital substances almost without loss, have a pleasant aroma and are suitable for a healthy kitchen.

Spices

The Mediterranean Diet count lots of selected spices that emphasize the taste of the dish, stimulate the appetite and the production of digestive juices, and improve the digestibility and utilization of food. Use them in right quantities, and with a sensitive stomach, it is better to completely abandon the exotic ones! To spices from local herbs, as a rule, there are no such complaints, and it is allowed to use everything that seems to smell delicious!

Fresh Greens

Fresh herbs make the dishes exquisite to taste, in addition, have healing powers (many are used in traditional medicine). Therefore, fresh greenery is given an honorable place in a healthy diet. Sparing methods of cooking dishes from plant foods make it possible to appreciate its natural flavor, which becomes even more attractive due to greens and spices.

Always give preference to fresh spicy greens, rather than dried. It would be a wish, and you can always grow your favorite grass in a flowerpot! Especially suitable for cultivation on the windowsill or in the garden are basil, savory, borage, dill, tarragon, chervil, lavage, marjoram, parsley, rosemary, onion, and garlic.

Fresh herbs (greens) have several advantages in comparison with dried herbs:

•   Herbs contain aromatic substances that emphasize the typical taste of the dish, and if used correctly, you can get a variety of taste options. Meals with greens, therefore, seem more delicious.

•   Dishes in which greens are added require less salt. When you eat bread, cheese, sausage, the salt hidden in them enters the body, the amount of which cannot be reduced. However, if you season your self-cooked dishes with herbs, no additional salting is required! You will be able to feel for yourself that dishes that do not contain any grains of table salt taste pleasantly salted.

• Dishes seasoned with herbs increase appetite and are easier to digest: the essential oils in herbs contribute to the secretion of digestive juices and better digestion of food.

Dried spices must be stored in an airtight and protected from light containers—preferably in a glass.

Sauces

For raw plant foods, vegetables, fish, sauces are used as seasonings. For salads, raw vegetable food, it is best to use exclusively olive oil and avoid totally purchased sauces for salads or mayonnaise!

If vegetable products undergo heat treatment—heating, cooking, then use juice produced during the cooking process or the water in which the heat treatment was performed as the basis of the sauce. Thickening should be done with flour dried in a dry pan, and other additives are not recommended. You can use the water in which the heat treatment of vegetable raw materials was used as the basis of any soup—this is very useful and tasty.

All commercially prepared broths, sauces, and soups cannot be part of a Mediterranean diet since they are concentrated, denatured and often very salted products.

Salt

Despite convincing explanations of the negative role of over-consumption of table salt for health, it still occupies a leading place in modern nutrition. Some people, even without trying the proposed dish, immediately grab the saltshaker and begin to shake it vigorously over the plate. Of course, salt is necessary as a mineral substance to ensure the vital activity of the organism, but its daily need is only 2-3 grams! Since such a quantity of sodium chloride—salt—is already contained in vegetable products, it is unnecessary in principle to salt food in addition. However, this is in theory, and in fact, our compatriots add 12–15 grams of salt daily to food for taste. As a result, the kidneys, which should remove excess, are heavily loaded, which is then fraught with diseases.

Therefore, every day you should control the amount of salt and not exceed 5-7 g. Healthy kidneys can cope with so much salt without damage to health. However, when the tongue gets used to lightly salted food, then you can again enjoy the real, your own, taste, characteristic of this or that dish, which previously "killed" excessive salt.

The Drinks

The body of an adult almost 70% consists of water; water-salt metabolism is continuously carried out in it. Therefore, the process of fluid intake is a key process in a healthy diet. A person can go hungry for weeks, but without water, the body can last only a few days.

How Much Should You Drink?

Daily fluid intake is at least 1.5–2 liters daily. This corresponds to 12–16 cups or 10–20 glasses of beverages. Try to control yourself: how much liquid do you drink during the day? If less than recommended, then this is, as they say, information for reflection!

Bodyweight (kg)	Daily minimum fluid requirement (l)
Up to 50	2.0
Up to 75	2.5
Up to 90	3.0
Over 90	Over 3.0

Moreover, two liters during the day is a general recommendation, and the individual need for health can be much higher. If the weather is hot and the person is sweating more than usual, then the need for fluid for him (or her) is much higher. With a large body mass and intense physical activity, the body's fluid supply should also be more than recommended. Do not be afraid of "overdose", however, if you suffer from progressive renal or cardiac weakness. In this case, you should follow the recommendations of the doctor on the daily intake of fluid.

Often this argument sounds like "I drink when I want, so this should be enough." Unfortunately, such an argument does not have a good reason: the feeling of thirst is a bad signal because it comes rather late. When there is thirst, the fluid balance is already shifted far beyond the danger zone. That is, thirst must be warned! It should also be borne in mind that older people are less likely to feel thirsty than younger people, the signal from the body is almost unheard of, so they should control the amount of fluid consumed.

However, the body's task is not only to consume the liquid, but also to drain it. Therefore, if you are satisfied with the average rate of daily fluid intake of 2 liters and you feel comfortable, then the body should eject 2 liters of light urine daily. This is good proof that your fluid balance is in excellent condition.

When Should You Drink?

Not only the amount but also the time of fluid intake is of great importance. Contrary to the widely ingrained tradition, one should drink a lot not during meals, but mainly between meals. There is quite a convincing reason for this: if you drink a lot with food, the water greatly dilutes digestive juices, which is why food stays in the stomach for a long time not properly processed.

It is necessary to drink half an hour before meals and not earlier than half an hour after the meal, but never during meals.

What Should I Drink?

The partial need for liquids is covered by water contained mainly in raw food, and approximately 1.5–2 liters per day (depending on temperature and physical activity) should be obtained by drinking beverages (water).

Pay attention to the quality of drinking water, knowing that from the water supply it is suitable for consumption only conditionally. With the introduction of chlorination of drinking water in the United States in the 20s of the last century, the level of thrombosis there, as calculated by scientists, increased 5 times! If it is not possible to purchase 2 liters of quality drinking water daily, then it is advisable to pour tap water into a container (preferably a glass) and stand it for 12 hours, stirring occasionally to remove chlorine. The same goal can be achieved by boiling water, for example for making tea. To some extent, the problem is also removed with the installation of a water filter. Choose the most reliable. Naturally, though, instead of tap water, natural water from proven sources is recommended.

When choosing mineral water, one should pay attention to its composition, which must be indicated on the label. Some contain a lot of sodium chloride (table salt) and nitrates, which makes them unsuitable for regular consumption. In addition, mineral waters should not contain large amounts of carbon dioxide—give preference to "calm" water.

It is good to use natural (without sugar, preservatives and other additives) fruit and vegetable juices and juices from fresh greens for drinking. You can make them yourself or buy them in specialized diet stores that guarantee good biological quality. Try different juices, as well as in this variety is welcome.

Milk as a liquid requirement is recommended only in small quantities (for adults no more than 1/4 l daily). It is better to try to enter into the diet of liquid dairy products, such as whey, low-Fat yogurt, buttermilk.

Herbal Teas

Warm drinks can be consumed in larger volumes than cold ones. Therefore, herbal teas are well established as a means to quench thirst. The benefits of herbal teas are beyond doubt, but caution is appropriate: many of them are medicinal and not intended for regular long-term consumption. If you do not suffer from high acidity, you can safely enjoy herbal tea, which contains, among other things, a lot of vitamin C and thoroughly washes the kidneys (prevention of kidney stones).

As with all remedies, for herbal teas the dose is crucial. It is possible to switch from one herbal tea to another for 1-2 weeks. If there is a desire to drink any of them for a long time, then first consult with your doctor. Only in the case of chronic illness, herbal tea is drunk for a long time, but again, only on the recommendation of a doctor!

Although herbal teas have healing properties, they should not taste like medicines. As an alternative to coffee in the morning, rosemary tea has proven itself very well, especially with low blood pressure. It awakens vitality and quickly activates blood circulation without causing side effects.

Teas made from a mixture of herbs are alkaline drinks, due to which they can liquefy excess acids or neutralize them additionally. In addition, stimulating the metabolism, they play a big role in the disinfection and elimination of toxins from the body.

If you do not have the opportunity to independently collect and dry herbs for teas, then you can buy them in a pharmacy, but not in supermarkets and certainly not from random sellers in the market, where the quality of collection and drying is not guaranteed.

Pour 1 teaspoon of the herbal mixture with 1 liter of boiling water; let it stand for 3-4 minutes, then strain the tea. In this way, you deliberately brew light, "liquid" tea that retains a magnificent aroma and provides the body with water without causing adverse reactions that can occur at higher concentrations (for example, cramps in the digestive tract).

Drinks are a Delight

For healthy people, in principle, there is no objection to coffee and black tea (1-2 cups daily, and coffee is better with milk) or light alcoholic beverages—beer, wine, and champagne. Some studies suggest that a moderate intake of red wine can help lower the risk of heart disease, and the Mediterranean diet encourages wine consumption (up to five ounces per day for women under the age of sixty-five and ten ounces for men under the age of sixty-five). Here it is appropriate to recall the words of the great Paracelsus that only the dose makes the substance non-toxic. Anyone who regularly drinks one cup of coffee with milk or a cup of not very strong black tea in the mornings and a small glass of wine or beer to relax in the evenings is unlikely to cause any harm to their health. The proportion of risk is significantly increased with excessive use.

Breakfast Recipes

1.   Morning Egg Sandwiches

Servings: 4

Preparation Time: 10 minutes

Cooking Time: 10 minutes

Ingredients

5 oz whole grain bread

1 tablespoon sunflower seeds butter

¼ teaspoon salt

1 avocado, pitted

4 eggs

Directions:

Slice the bread into 8 slices.

Preheat a skillet and add the sunflower seeds butter and melt it well.

Beat the eggs in the skillet and sprinkle them with the salt.

Chop the avocado into the medium cubes and mash it well.

Spread the bread slices with the avocado mash.

When the eggs are cooked, cool them a little and place on top of the bread slices to make the sandwiches.

Serve the dish immediately.

Nutrition: calories: 275,

Fat: 17.7g, total Carbs: 21.7g,

sugars: 3.2g, Protein: 11.1g

2.   Quinoa Bowl

Servings: 6

Preparation Time: 10 minutes

Cooking Time: 15 minutes

Ingredients

2 cups quinoa

1 cup blueberries

1 cup coconut milk, unsweetened

2 cups water

2 tablespoons almonds

1 teaspoon pistachio

2 tablespoons honey

Directions:

Combine the coconut milk and water together in the saucepan and stir the liquid well.

Add the quinoa and close the lid.

Cook the mixture on medium heat for 5 minutes.

Wash the blueberries carefully and add them to the quinoa mixture.

Stir it carefully and continue to cook.

Combine the pistachio and almonds together and crush the nuts.

Sprinkle the quinoa with the crushed nuts and cook the mixture for 3 minutes more.

Add honey and stir the mixture carefully until honey has dissolved.

Transfer to serving bowls and enjoy.

 Enjoy!

Nutrition:

Calories: 348, Fat: 14.1g,

Total Carbs: 48.3g,

Sugars: 9.6g, Protein: 9.6g

3.   Sweet Oatmeal

Servings: 3

Preparation Time: 5 minutes

Cooking Time: 10 minutes

Ingredients

1 cup oatmeal

5 apricots

1 tablespoon honey

1 cup coconut milk, unsweetened

1 teaspoon cashew butter

¼ teaspoon salt

½ cup water

Directions:

Combine the coconut milk and oatmeal together in the saucepan and stir the mixture.

Add the water and stir it again. Sprinkle the mixture with the salt and close the lid.

Cook the oatmeal on medium heat for 10 minutes.

Meanwhile, chop the apricots into tiny pieces and combine the chopped fruit with the honey.

When the oatmeal is cooked, add cashew butter and fruit mixture.

Stir carefully and transfer to serving bowls.

Serve immediately.

Nutrition:

Calories: 336,

Fat: 21.2g,

Total Carbs: 35.1g,

Sugars: 14.0g,

Protein: 6.2g

4. Green Beans and Eggs

Servings: 2

Preparation Time: 10 minutes

Cooking Time: 15 minutes

Ingredients

½ cup green beans

¼ teaspoon salt

5 eggs

1/3 cup skim milk

1 bell pepper, seeds removed

1 teaspoon olive oil

Directions:

Slice the bell pepper and combine it with the green beans.

Pour the olive oil in a skillet and transfer the vegetable mixture to the skillet.

Cook on medium heat for 3 minutes, stirring frequently.

Meanwhile, beat the eggs in a mixing bowl.

Sprinkle the egg mixture with the salt and add skim milk. Whisk well.

Pour the egg mixture over the vegetable mixture and cook for 3 minutes on medium heat.

Stir the mixture carefully so that the eggs and vegetables are well combined.

Cook for 4 minutes more.

Stir again and close the lid.

Cook the scrambled eggs for 5 minutes more.

Stir the mixture again.

Serve it.

Nutrition:

Calories: 231,

Fat: 13.4g,

Total Carbs: 9.3g,

Sugars: 6.2g,

Protein: 16.3g

5.   Spiced Morning Omelet

Servings: 3

Preparation Time: 10 minutes

Cooking Time: 15 minutes

Ingredients

7 eggs

1/3 cup skim milk

3 garlic cloves

¼ teaspoon nutmeg

¼ teaspoon ground ginger

1 teaspoon cilantro

1 teaspoon olive oil

1 tablespoon chives

1 teaspoon turmeric

Directions:

Beat the eggs in a mixing bowl.

Add the skim milk and whisk again.

Sprinkle the egg mixture with the nutmeg, ground ginger, cilantro, and turmeric.

Peel the garlic cloves and mince them.

Chop the chives and combine with the minced garlic.

Add the herb mixture to the eggs and stir it again.

Preheat a skillet well and pour in the olive oil.

Preheat the olive oil over medium heat and then pour the egg mixture into the pan.

Close the lid and cook the omelet for 15 minutes.

When the dish is cooked, cool slightly and cut into the serving portions.

Serve it.

Nutrition:

Calories: 179,

Fat: 12.0g,

Total Carbs: 3.8g,

Sugars: 2.2g,

Protein: 14.1g

## 6.	Rice Pudding

Servings: 5

Preparation Time: 5 minutes

Cooking Time: 15 minutes

Ingredients

1 cup brown rice

2 cups coconut milk, unsweetened

1 teaspoon cinnamon

1 teaspoon ginger

1/3 teaspoon thyme

1/3 cup almonds

2 tablespoon honey

1 teaspoon lemon zest

Directions:

Pour the coconut milk into a saucepan and heat over medium.

Add the brown rice and stir the mixture carefully.

Close the lid and cook the brown rice over medium heat for 10 minutes.

Meanwhile, crush the almonds and combine them with the lemon zest, thyme, ginger, and cinnamon.

Sprinkle the brown rice with the almond mixture and stir it carefully.

Close the lid and cook the dish for 5 minutes.

When the pudding is cooked, remove it from the saucepan and transfer to a big bowl.

Add the honey and stir the pudding.

Serve it immediately.

Nutrition:

Calories: 423,

Fat: 27.1g,

Total Carbs: 43.3g,

Sugars: 10.4g,

Protein: 6.5g

7. Creamy Millet

Servings: 8

Preparation Time: 10 minutes

Cooking Time: 15 minutes

Ingredients

2 cups millet

1 cup almond milk, unsweetened

1 cup water

1 cup coconut milk, unsweetened

1 teaspoon cinnamon

½ teaspoon ground ginger

¼ teaspoon salt

1 tablespoon chia seeds

1 tablespoon cashew butter

4 oz Parmesan cheese, grated

Directions:

Combine the coconut milk, almond milk, and water together in the saucepan.

Stir the liquid gently and add millet.

Mix carefully and close the lid.

Cook the millet on the medium heat for 5 minutes.

Sprinkle the porridge with the cinnamon, ground ginger, salt, and chia seeds.

Stir the mixture carefully with a spoon and continue to cook on medium heat for 5 minutes more.

Add the cashew butter and cook the millet for 5 minutes.

Remove the millet from the heat and transfer it to serving bowls.

Sprinkle the dish with the grated cheese.

Serve it.

Nutrition:

Calories: 384,

Fat: 19.8g,

Total Carbs: 42.9g,

Sugars: 3.6g,

Protein: 11.7g

8.   Apple muffins

Servings: 5

Preparation Time: 10 minutes

Cooking Time: 15 minutes

Ingredients

2 eggs

1 cup oat flour

½ teaspoon salt

2 tablespoon stevia

3 apples, washed and peeled

½ cup skim milk

1 tablespoon olive oil

½ teaspoon baking soda

1 teaspoon apple cider vinegar

Directions:

Beat the eggs in the mixing bowl and whisk them well.

Add the skim milk, salt, baking soda, stevia, and apple cider vinegar.

Stir the mixture carefully.

Grate the apples and add the grated mixture in the egg mixture.

Stir it carefully and add the oat flour.

Add the olive oil and blend into a smooth batter

Preheat the oven to 350 F.

Fill each muffin form halfway with the batter and place the muffins in the oven.

Cook the dish for 15 minutes.

Remove the cooked muffins from the oven.

Cool the cooked muffins well and serve them.

Nutrition:

Calories: 200,

Fat: 6.0g,

Total Carbs: 32.4g,

Sugars: 15.3g,

Protein: 11.7g

9.   Mushroom Frittata

Servings: 5

Preparation Time: 10 minutes

Cooking Time: 20 minutes

Ingredients

8 oz shiitake mushrooms

1 teaspoon salt

1 cup broccoli

7 eggs

5 oz Parmesan cheese

1 tablespoon olive oil

½ teaspoon ground ginger

5 garlic cloves

1 teaspoon oregano

1 teaspoon basil

1 teaspoon cilantro

½ cup low-

Fat milk

Directions:

Wash the shiitake mushrooms well and chop them.

Chop the broccoli and combine it with the mushrooms in a mixing bowl.

In a separate bowl, beat the eggs.

Sprinkle the egg mixture with the cilantro, basil, oregano, and ground ginger. Stir it well.

Add the low-Fat milk and broccoli. Stir the egg mixture well.

Peel the garlic cloves and mince them.

Add minced garlic in the egg mixture and stir it gently.

Preheat the oven to 350 F.

Spray a deep pan with olive oil

Pour the egg mixture into the pan and place it in the preheated oven.

Cook the frittata for 20 minutes.

When the dish is cooked, remove it from the oven and cool slightly.

Serve the frittata immediately.

Nutrition:

Calories: 250,

Fat: 15.5g,

Total Carbs: 11.5g,

Sugars: 3.7g,

Protein: 19.2g

10. Homemade Granola Bowl

Servings: 6

Preparation Time: 10 minutes

Cooking Time: 20 minutes

Ingredients

3 tablespoons pumpkin seeds

1 tablespoon coconut oil

1 teaspoon sunflower seeds

¼ cup almonds

1 cup raw oats

3 tablespoons sesame seeds

5 tablespoons honey

2 cups almond milk, unsweetened

Directions:

Combine the pumpkin seeds, sunflower seeds, almonds, and sesame seeds together.

Crush the mixture well and add raw oats.

Add the honey and coconut oil.

Stir the mixture carefully until you get a smooth mix.

Preheat the oven to 350 F.

Cover the tray with parchment and transfer the seed mixture onto the tray. Flatten it well.

Put the tray in the preheated oven and cook it for 20 minutes.

When the mixture is cooked, remove it from the oven and chill well.

Separate the mixture into small pieces and put in serving bowls.

Add the almond milk and mix up the dish.

Serve it.

Nutrition:

Calories: 381,

Fat: 28.5g,

Total Carbs: 30.8g,

Sugars: 17.4g,

Protein: 6.4g

11. Breakfast Kale Frittata

Preparation time: 10 minutes

Cooking time: 30 minutes

Servings: 4

Ingredients:

6 kale stalks, chopped

1 small sweet onion, chopped

1 small broccoli head, florets separated

2 garlic cloves, minced

Salt and black pepper to the taste

4 eggs

1 tablespoon olive oil

Directions:

Heat up a pan with the oil over medium-high heat, add the onion, stir and cook for 4-5 minutes. Add the garlic, broccoli and kale, toss and cook for 5 minutes more. Add the eggs, salt and pepper and mix. Place in the oven and bake at 380 degrees F for 20 minutes. Slice and serve for breakfast.

Enjoy!

Nutrition:

Calories 214,

Fat 7,

Fiber 2,

Carbs 12,

Protein 8

12. Cranberry Granola Bars

Preparation time: 2 hours

Cooking time: 0 minutes

Servings: 4

Ingredients:

2 cups walnuts, toasted

1 cup dates, pitted

3 tablespoons water

¾ cup cranberries, dried, no added sugar

2 cups desiccated coconut, unsweetened

Directions:

In your food processor, mix dates with coconut, cranberries, water and walnuts. Pulse well then spread the mix into a lined baking dish. Press well into the dish and keep in the fridge for 2 hours then cut into bars and serve. Enjoy!

Nutrition: Calories 476, Fat 40,

Fiber 9, Carbs 33, Protein 6

13. Spinach and Berry Smoothie

Preparation time: 10 minutes

Cooking time: 0 minutes

Servings: 2

Ingredients:

1 cup blackberries

1 avocado, pitted, peeled and chopped

1 banana, peeled and roughly chopped

1 cup baby spinach

1 tablespoon hemp seeds

1 cup water

½ cup almond milk, unsweetened

Directions:

In your blender, mix the berries with the avocado, banana, spinach, hemp seeds, water and almond milk. Pulse well, divide into 2 glasses and serve for breakfast. Enjoy!

Nutrition: Calories 160, Fat 3, Fiber 4,

Carbs 6, Protein 3

14.   Zucchini Breakfast Salad

Preparation time: 10 minutes

Cooking time: 0 minutes

Servings: 4

Ingredients: 2 zucchinis, spiralized

1 cup beets, baked, peeled and grated

½ bunch kale, chopped

2 tablespoons olive oil

For the tahini sauce:

1 tablespoon maple syrup

Juice of 1 lime

¼ inch fresh ginger, grated

1/3 cup sesame seed paste

Directions:

In a salad bowl, mix the zucchinis with the beets, kale and oil. In another small bowl, whisk the maple syrup with lime juice, ginger and sesame paste. Pour the dressing over the salad, toss and serve it for breakfast. Enjoy!

Nutrition: Calories 183, Fat 3, Fiber 2,

Carbs 7,

Protein 9

15.   Quinoa and Spinach Breakfast Salad

Preparation time: 10 minutes

Cooking time: 0 minutes

Servings: 2

Ingredients: 16 ounces quinoa, cooked

1 handful raisins

1 handful baby spinach leaves

1 tablespoon maple syrup

½ tablespoon lemon juice

4 tablespoons olive oil

1 teaspoon ground cumin

A pinch of sea salt and black pepper

½ teaspoon chili flakes

Directions: In a bowl, mix the quinoa with the spinach, raisins, cumin, salt and pepper and toss. Add the maple syrup, lemon juice, oil and chili flakes and toss then serve for breakfast. Enjoy!

Nutrition: Calories 170, Fat 3, Fiber 6,

Carbs 8,

Protein 5

222

16. Carrots Breakfast Mix

Preparation time: 10 minutes

Cooking time: 0 minutes

Servings: 4

Ingredients: 1½ tablespoon maple syrup

1 teaspoon olive oil

1 tablespoon chopped walnuts

1 onion, chopped   4 cups shredded carrots

1 tablespoon curry powder

¼ teaspoon ground turmeric

Black pepper to the taste

2 tablespoons sesame seed paste

¼ cup lemon juice   ½ cup chopped parsley

Directions:

In a salad bowl, mix the onion with the carrots, turmeric, curry powder, black pepper, lemon juice and parsley. Add the maple syrup, oil, walnuts and sesame seed paste. toss well and serve for breakfast. Enjoy!

Nutrition: Calories 150, Fat 3,

Fiber 2, Carbs 6, Protein 8

17. Italian Breakfast Salad

Preparation time: 10 minutes

Cooking time: 0 minutes

Servings: 4

Ingredients:

1 handful kalamata olives, pitted and sliced

1 cup cherry tomatoes, halved

1½ cucumbers, sliced

1 red onion, chopped

2 tablespoons chopped oregano

1 tablespoon chopped mint

For the salad dressing:

2 tablespoons balsamic vinegar

¼ cup olive oil

1 garlic clove, minced

2 teaspoons dried Italian herbs

A pinch of salt and black pepper

Directions:

In a salad bowl, toss together the olives with the tomatoes, cucumbers, onion, mint and oregano. In a smaller bowl, whisk the vinegar with the oil, garlic, Italian herbs, salt and pepper. Pour the dressing over the salad, toss and serve for breakfast. Enjoy!

Nutrition: Calories 191, Fat 10,

Fiber 3, Carbs 13, Protein 1

18.   Zucchini and Sprout Breakfast Mix

Preparation time: 10 minutes

Cooking time: 0 minutes

Servings: 4

Ingredients:

2 zucchinis, spiralized

2 cups bean sprouts

4 green onions, chopped

1 red bell pepper, chopped

Juice of 1 lime

1 tablespoon olive oil

½ cup chopped cilantro

¾ cup almonds chopped

A pinch of salt and black pepper

Directions:

In a salad bowl, toss together the zucchinis with the bean sprouts, green onions, bell pepper, cilantro, almonds, salt, pepper, lime juice and oil. Serve for breakfast.

Nutrition: Calories 140, Fat 4, Fiber 2,

Carbs 7, Protein 8

19.   Breakfast Corn Salad

Preparation time: 10 minutes

Cooking time: 0 minutes

Servings: 4

Ingredients:

2 avocados, pitted, peeled and cubed

1-pint mixed cherry tomatoes, halved

2 cups fresh corn kernels

1 red onion, chopped

For the salad dressing:

2 tablespoons olive oil

1 tablespoon lime juice

½ teaspoon grated lime zest

A pinch of salt and black pepper

¼ cup chopped cilantro

Directions:

In a salad bowl, mix the avocados with the tomatoes, corn and onion. Add the oil, lime juice, lime zest, salt, pepper and the cilantro, toss and serve for breakfast.

Nutrition: Calories 140, Fat 3, Fiber 2, Carbs 6, Protein 9

1 garlic clove, minced

1 bunch basil, roughly chopped

Directions:

In a salad bowl, toss together the cucumber with the tomatoes, onion, salt, pepper, oil, vinegar, basil and garlic. Serve for breakfast.

Enjoy!

Nutrition: Calories 100, Fat 1, Fiber 2, Carbs 2, Protein 6

20.   Simple Basil Tomato Mix

Preparation time: 10 minutes

Cooking time: 0 minutes

Servings: 6

Ingredients:

½ cup extra-virgin olive oil

1 cucumber, chopped

2 pints colored cherry tomatoes, halved

Salt and black pepper to the taste

1 red onion, chopped

3 tablespoons red vinegar

21.   Cucumber and Avocado Salad

Preparation time: 10 minutes

Cooking time: 0 minutes

Servings: 4

Ingredients:

1-pound cucumbers, chopped

2 avocados, pitted and chopped

1 small red onion, thinly sliced

2 tablespoons olive oil

2 tablespoons lemon juice

¼ cup chopped parsley

A pinch of salt and black pepper

Directions:

In a salad bowl, mix the cucumbers with the avocados, onion, oil, lemon juice, parsley, salt and pepper. Serve for breakfast.

Enjoy!

Nutrition: Calories 120, Fat 2,

Fiber 2, Carbs 3, Protein 4

22.   Watermelon Salad

Preparation time: 10 minutes

Cooking time: 0 minutes

Servings: 2

Ingredients:

½ teaspoon agave nectar

2 tablespoons lemon juice

1 tablespoon extra-virgin olive oil

1 jalapeno, seeded and chopped

12 ounces watermelon, chopped

1 red onion, thinly sliced

½ cup chopped basil leaves

2 cups baby arugula

Directions:

In a bowl, toss together the watermelon with the jalapeno, onion, basil, arugula, oil, agave nectar, lemon juice and oil. Serve for breakfast.

Nutrition: Calories 128, Fat 8, Fiber 2,

Carbs 16, Protein 2

Lunch recipes

23.   Falafel bowls with tahini sauce

Preparation Time: 20 minutes

Cooking Time: 20 minutes

Servings: 4

Ingredients:

One package or eight ounces of frozen prepared falafel

A two-thirds cup of water

Half cup of whole-wheat couscous

One bag or sixteen ounces of fresh and steam-in-bag green beans

Half cup of Tahini Sauce

Half cup of pitted Kalamata olives

One-fourth cup of crumbled feta cheese

Directions:

Bring water in a saucepan and stir in couscous.

Cover and then remove it from the heat.

Allow standing until you see the liquid getting absorbed. Wait for five minutes. After which, fluff with a fork and set aside.

Now, prepare the green beans and tahini sauce.

Divide the portion among four small containers and refrigerate.

Divide green beans among four serving containers.

Top every container with half cup couscous, 1/4th falafel, and one tsp. of olives and feta.

Refrigerate for four days after sealing it.

While serving, reheat it in a microwave for two minutes.

Right before eating, garnish it with tahini sauce.

Nutrition: Calories: 500 Protein: 15 G

Fat: 727G Carbs: 55 G

24.   Spinach and egg scramble with raspberries

Preparation Time: 10 minutes

Cooking Time: 10 minutes

Servings: 1

Ingredients:

One teaspoon of canola oil

One and a half cups of baby spinach (which is one and a half ounces)

Two eggs, large and lightly beaten

Kosher salt, a pinch.

ground pepper, a pinch

One slice of whole-grain toasted bread

Half cup of fresh and fine raspberries

Directions:

Heat the oil in a non-stick and small skillet at a temperature of medium-high.

Add spinach to the plate.

Cleanly wipe the pan and add eggs into the medium heated pan.

Stir and cook twice in order to ensure even-cooking for about two minutes.

Stir the spinach in and add salt and pepper into it.

Garnish it with raspberries and toast before eating.

Nutrition: Calories: 296 rotein: 18 G

Fat: 16 G Carbs: 21 G

25.   Mediterranean lettuce wraps

Preparation Time: 10 minutes

Cooking Time: 10 minutes

Servings: 3

Ingredients:

One-fourth cup of tahini

One-fourth cup of olive oil, extra-virgin

One teaspoon of lemon zest

One-fourth cup of lemon juice

One and a half tsp. of pure maple syrup

Three fourth tsp. of kosher salt

Half tsp. of paprika

Two cans (15 ounces) of rinsed chickpeas, no-salt-added

Half cup of sliced and roasted red pepper - drained and jarred

Half cup of thinly sliced shallots

Twelve leaves of Bibb lettuce, large

One-fourth cup of almonds, roasted and chopped

Two tsp. of fresh parsley, chopped

Directions:

Whisk lemon zest, tahini, oil, maple syrup, lemon juice, paprika, and all in a bowl.

After which, add peppers, chickpeas, and shallots.

Now, toss for coating.

After this, divide this mixture among the lettuce leaves (say about one-third cup for every portion).

Top with parsley and almonds.

Before serving, wrap lettuce leaves around this filling for proper garnishing.

Nutrition: Calories: 498 Protein: 16 G

Fat: 28 G Carbs: 44 G

26. Pressed Tuna Sandwich

Preparation Time: 40 minutes

Cooking Time: 2 hours and 40 minutes

Servings: 4

Ingredients:

Half cup of red onion, thinly sliced

Five tsp. of divided red-wine vinegar, divided

Two tsp. of boiling water

A twelve inch of the crusty country loaf, whole-wheat should be taken about one pound

Two tsp. of olive oil, extra-virgin

One tsp. of Dijon mustard

Half tsp. of pepper, ground

One-fourth tsp. of salt

Two cans or five ounces of chunk and drained light tuna, oil-packed

One cup of baby arugula, packed

One cup of English cucumber, thinly sliced

One cup of radishes, thinly sliced

One cup of quartered cherry tomatoes

Half cup of olives pitted and unevenly chopped

Four thinly sliced boiled eggs, hard and large

One-fourth cup of fresh basil, packed

Directions:

Combine two tsp. of vinegar, water, and onions into one small bowl.

Marinate and stir for ten minutes.

Cut horizontal loaves in half.

Pull out inner bread from the halves by leaving around half an inch.

Whisk three tsp of vinegar, oil, pepper, salt, and mustard in one bowl.

Drain the onion and add arugula, tuna, radishes, cucumber, olives, and tomatoes.

Stuff the mixture into the bottom half of one loaf.

Top with basil, eggs, and the loaf's top.

Refrigerate for two hours.

Nutrition: Calories: 266 Protein: 13 G

Fat: 12 G Carbs: 23 G

27. Cauliflower Soup

Preparation Time: 10 minutes

Cooking Time: 50 minutes

Servings: 4

Ingredients:

3 pounds cauliflower, florets separated

1 yellow onion, chopped

1 tablespoon coconut oil

Black pepper to the taste

2 garlic cloves, minced

2 carrots, chopped

2 cups beef stock

1 cup water

½ cup coconut milk

1 teaspoon olive oil

2 tablespoons parsley, chopped

Directions:

Heat up a pot with the coconut oil over medium-high heat, add carrots, onion and garlic, stir and cook for 5 minutes.

Add cauliflower, water and stock, stir, bring to a boil, cover and cook for 45 minutes.

Transfer soup to your blender and pulse well, add coconut milk, pulse well again, ladle into bowls, drizzle the olive oil over the soup, sprinkle parsley and serve for lunch.

Nutrition: Calories: 190 Protein: 4 G

Fat: 2 G Carbs: 16 G

28.   Purple Potato Soup

Preparation Time: 10 minutes

Cooking Time: 1 hour and 15 minutes

Servings: 6

Ingredients: 6 purple potatoes, chopped

1 cauliflower head, florets separated

Black pepper to the taste

4 garlic cloves, minced

1 yellow onion, chopped

3 tablespoons olive oil

1 tablespoon thyme, chopped

1 leek, chopped

2 shallots, chopped

4 cups chicken stock, low-sodium

Directions:

In a baking dish, mix potatoes with onion, cauliflower, garlic, pepper, thyme and half of the oil, toss to coat, introduce in the oven and bake for 45 minutes at 400 degrees F.

Heat up a pot with the rest of the oil over medium-high heat, add leeks and shallots, stir and cook for 10 minutes.

Add roasted veggies and stock, stir, bring to a boil, cook for 20 minutes, transfer soup to your food processor, blend well, divide into bowls and serve.

Nutrition: Calories: 200 Protein: 8 G

Fat: 8 G Carbs: 15 G

29.   Broccoli Soup

Preparation Time: 10 minutes

Cooking Time: 1 hour

Servings: 4

Ingredients:

2 pounds broccoli, florets separated

1 yellow onion, chopped

1 tablespoon olive oil

Black pepper to the taste

1 cup celery, chopped   2 carrots, chopped

3 and ½ cups low-sodium chicken stock

1 tablespoon cilantro chopped

Directions: Heat up a pot with the oil over medium-high heat, add the onion, celery and carrots, stir and cook for 5 minutes.   Add broccoli, black pepper and stock, stir and cook over medium heat for 1 hour.

Pulse using an immersion blender, add cilantro, stir the soup again, divide into bowls and serve.

Nutrition: Calories: 170   Protein: 9 G

Fat: 2 G   Carbs: 10 G

30.   Leeks Soup

Preparation Time: 10 minutes

Cooking Time: 1 hour and 15 minutes

Servings: 6

Ingredients:

2 gold potatoes, chopped

1 cup cauliflower florets

Black pepper to the taste

5 leeks, chopped

4 garlic cloves, minced

1 yellow onion, chopped

3 tablespoons olive oil

A handful parsley, chopped

4 cups low-sodium chicken stock

Directions:

Heat up a pot with the oil over medium-high heat, add onion and garlic, stir and cook for 5 minutes.

Add potatoes, cauliflower, black pepper, leeks and stock, stir, bring to a simmer, cook over medium heat for 30 minutes, blend using an immersion blender, add parsley, stir, ladle into bowls and serve.

Nutrition: Calories: 150 Protein: 8 G

Fat: 8 G Carbs: 7 G

31.   Cauliflower Lunch Salad

Preparation Time: 2 hours

Cooking Time: 10 minutes

Servings: 4

Ingredients:

1/3 cup low-sodium veggie stock

2 tablespoons olive oil

6 cups cauliflower florets, grated

Black pepper to the taste

¼ cup red onion, chopped

1 red bell pepper, chopped

Juice of ½ lemon

½ cup kalamata olives, pitted and cut into halves

1 teaspoon mint, chopped

1 tablespoon cilantro, chopped

Directions:

Heat up a pan with the oil over medium-high heat, add cauliflower, pepper and stock, stir, cook for 10 minutes, transfer to a bowl and keep in the fridge for 2 hours.

Mix cauliflower with olives, onion, bell pepper, black pepper, mint, cilantro and lemon juice, toss to coat and serve.

Nutrition: Calories: 185 Protein: 8 G

Fat: 12 G Carbs: 11 G

32.   Shrimp Soup

Preparation Time: 10 minutes

Cooking Time: 15 minutes

Servings: 6

Ingredients:

46 ounces low-sodium chicken stock

3 cups shrimp, peeled and deveined

A pinch of black pepper

2 tablespoons green onions, chopped

1 teaspoon dill, chopped

Directions:

Put the stock in a pot, bring to a simmer over medium heat, add black pepper, onion and shrimp, stir and simmer for 8-10 minutes.

Add dill, stir, cook for 5 minutes more, ladle into bowls and serve.

Nutrition: Calories: 190 Protein: 8 G

Fat: 7 G Carbs: 12 G

33.   Shrimp Mix

Preparation Time: 10 minutes

Cooking Time: 10 minutes

Servings: 4

Ingredients:

1 and ½ pounds shrimp, peeled and deveined

1 tablespoon olive oil

1 teaspoon sesame seeds

24 ounces broccoli florets

1 green onion, chopped

1 tablespoon balsamic vinegar

2 garlic cloves, minced

1 tablespoon ginger, grated

Directions:

In a bowl, mix oil with vinegar, garlic and ginger and whisk.

Transfer this to a pan, heat up over medium heat, add shrimp, stir and cook for 3 minutes.

Add broccoli, stir, cook for 4 minutes more,

Add sesame seeds and green onions, toss, divide everything between plates and serve.

Nutrition: Calories: 265 Protein: 20 G

Fat: 2 G Carbs: 10 G

34.   Spinach And Lentils Stew

Preparation Time: 10 minutes

Cooking Time: 23 minutes

Servings: 3

Ingredients:

1 teaspoon olive oil

1/3 cup brown lentils

1 teaspoon ginger, grated

4 garlic cloves, minced

1 green chili pepper, chopped

2 tomatoes, chopped

½ teaspoon turmeric powder

2 potatoes, cubed

A pinch of black pepper

¼ teaspoon cinnamon powder

1 cup low-sodium veggie stock

6 ounces spinach leaves

Directions:

Heat up a pot with the oil over medium heat, add chili pepper, ginger and garlic, stir and cook for 3 minutes.

Add tomatoes, pepper, cinnamon, turmeric, lentils, potatoes, stock and spinach, stir and cook for 20 minutes.

Divide into bowls and serve.

Nutrition: Calories: 220   Protein: 11 G

Fat: 3 G   Carbs: 16 G

35.   Sweet Potato Mix

Preparation Time: 10 minutes

Cooking Time: 25 minutes

Servings: 4

Ingredients:

1 small yellow onion, chopped

1 tablespoon olive oil

2 garlic cloves, minced

4 sweet potatoes, chopped

1 red bell pepper, chopped

14 ounces canned tomatoes, chopped

2 teaspoons curry powder

A pinch of black pepper

2 tablespoons red curry paste

14 ounces coconut milk

Juice of 3 limes

1 tablespoon cilantro, chopped

Directions:

Heat up a pot with the oil over medium heat, add onion, stir and cook for 5 minutes.

Add garlic, ginger, sweet potatoes, red bell pepper, tomatoes, curry powder, black pepper, curry paste, coconut milk, lime juice and cilantro, stir and simmer over medium heat for 20 minutes.

Divide into bowls and serve for lunch.

Nutrition: Calories: 270   Protein: 7 G

Fat: 7 G   Carbs: 12 G

36.   Pea Stew

Preparation Time: 10 minutes

Cooking Time: 25 minutes

Servings: 4

Ingredients:

1 carrot, cubed

1 yellow onion, chopped

1 and ½ tablespoons olive oil

1 celery stick, chopped

5 garlic cloves, minced

2 cups yellow peas

1 and ½ teaspoons cumin, ground

1 teaspoon sweet paprika

¼ teaspoon chili powder

A pinch of black pepper

¼ teaspoon cinnamon powder

½ cup tomatoes, chopped

Juice of ½ lemon

1-quart low-sodium veggie stock

1 tablespoon chives, chopped

Directions:

Heat up a pot with the oil over medium heat, add carrots, onion and celery, stir and cook for 5-6 minutes.

Add garlic, peas, cumin, paprika, chili powder, pepper, cinnamon, tomatoes, lemon juice, peas and stock, stir, bring to a simmer, cook over medium heat for 20 minutes, add chives, toss, divide into bowls and serve.

Nutrition: Calories: 272   Protein: 9 G

Fat: 6 G   Carbs: 14 G

37.   Green Beans Stew

Preparation Time: 10 minutes

Cooking Time: 25 minutes

Servings: 4

Ingredients: 2 tablespoons olive oil

2 carrots, chopped   1 yellow onion, chopped

20 ounces green beans

2 garlic cloves, minced

7 ounces canned tomatoes, chopped

5 cups low-sodium veggie stock

A pinch of black pepper

1 tablespoon parsley, chopped

Directions: Heat up a pot with the oil, over medium heat, add onion, stir and cook for 5 minutes.

Add carrots, green beans, garlic, tomatoes, black pepper and stock, stir, cover and simmer over medium heat for 20 minutes.

Add parsley, divide into bowls and serve for lunch.

Nutrition: Calories: 281   Protein: 11 G

Fat: 5 G   Carbs: 14 G

38.   Mushroom And Veggie Soup

Preparation Time: 10 minutes

Cooking Time: 25 minutes

Servings: 4

Ingredients:

1 yellow onion, chopped

A pinch of black pepper

1 tablespoon olive oil

1 red chili pepper, chopped

2 carrots, sliced

4 garlic cloves, minced

12 mushrooms, chopped

2 ounces kale leaves, roughly chopped

4 cups low-sodium veggie stock

1 cup tomatoes, chopped

½ tablespoon lemon zest, grated

½ tablespoon parsley, chopped

Directions:

Heat up a pot with the oil, over medium heat, add onion, garlic, chili and carrots, stir and sauté for 5 minutes.

Add black pepper, mushrooms, kale, tomatoes, stock and lemon zest, stir, cover and cook over medium heat for 20 minutes.

Add parsley, toss, divide into bowls and serve for lunch.

Nutrition: Calories: 200 Protein: 10 G

Fat: 6 G Carbs: 9 G

39. Jackfruit And Chili Stew

Preparation Time: 10 minutes

Cooking Time: 25 minutes

Servings: 4

Ingredients:

40 ounces canned jackfruit

14 ounces canned red chili puree

1 yellow onion, chopped

8 garlic cloves, minced

1 tablespoon olive oil

6 cups low-sodium veggie stock

1 tablespoon oregano, chopped

1 tablespoon cilantro, chopped

Directions:

Heat up a pot with the oil, over medium-high heat, add onion and garlic, stir and cook for 4-5 minutes.

Add jackfruit, chili puree and stock, stir, cover and cook over medium heat for 15 minutes.

Add oregano and cilantro, stir, cook for 5 minutes more, divide into bowls and serve.

Nutrition: Calories: 263 Protein: 11 G

Fat: 6 G Carbs: 13 G

40. Mushroom Lunch Salad

Preparation Time: 10 minutes

Cooking Time: 20 minutes

Servings: 4

Ingredients:

7 garlic cloves, minced

2 red chili peppers, chopped

1 teaspoon olive oil

1 yellow onion, chopped

1 teaspoon cumin, ground

½ teaspoon oregano, dried

½ teaspoon smoked paprika

A pinch of black pepper

¼ teaspoon cinnamon powder

1 cup low sodium veggie stock

8 ounces white mushrooms, sliced

3 teaspoons lime juice

Directions:

Heat up a pot with the oil over medium-high heat, add garlic and chili, stir and cook for 5 minutes.

Add onion, cumin, oregano, paprika, black pepper and cinnamon, stir and cook for 5 minutes.

Add mushrooms, lime juice and stock, stir, cook for 10 minutes, divide between plates and serve.

Nutrition: Calories: 221   Protein: 8 G

Fat: 6 G   Carbs: 12 G

41.   Chickpeas Stew

Preparation Time: 10 minutes

Cooking Time: 40 minutes

Servings: 4

Ingredients:

1 teaspoon olive oil

1 cup chickpeas, soaked for 8 hours and drained

4 garlic cloves, minced

1 yellow onion, chopped

1 green chili pepper, chopped

1 teaspoon coriander, ground

½ teaspoon cumin, ground

½ teaspoon sweet paprika

2 tomatoes, chopped

1 and ½ cups low-sodium veggie stock

A pinch of black pepper

3 cups spinach leaves

1 tablespoon lemon juice

Directions:

Heat up a pot with the oil over medium heat, add garlic, onion and chili pepper, stir and cook for 5 minutes.

Add coriander, cumin, paprika and black pepper, stir and cook for 5 minutes more.

Add chickpeas, tomatoes, stock and lemon juice, stir, cover the pot, cook over medium heat for 25 minutes, add spinach, cook for 5 minutes more, divide into bowls and serve.

Nutrition: Calories: 270

Protein: 9 G   Fat: 7 G   Carbs: 14 G

42.   Eggplant Stew

Preparation Time: 10 minutes

Cooking Time: 20 minutes

Servings: 4

Ingredients: ½ teaspoon cumin seeds

1 tablespoon coriander seeds

½ teaspoon mustard seeds

1 tablespoon olive oil

1 tablespoon ginger, grated

2 garlic cloves, minced

1 green chili pepper, chopped

A pinch of cinnamon powder

½ teaspoon cardamom, ground

½ teaspoon turmeric powder

1 teaspoon lime juice

4 baby eggplants, cubed

1 cup low-sodium veggie stock

1 tablespoon cilantro, chopped

Directions: Heat up a pot with the oil over medium-high heat, add cumin, coriander and mustard seeds, stir and cook them for 5 minutes.

Add ginger, garlic, chili, cinnamon, cardamom and turmeric, stir and cook for 5 minutes more.

Add lime juice, eggplants and stock, stir, cover and cook over medium heat for 15 minutes.   Add cilantro, stir, divide into bowls and serve for lunch.

Nutrition: Calories: 270   Protein: 9 G

Fat: 4 G Carbs: 12 G

43.   Black Eyed Peas Chili

Preparation Time: 10 minutes

Cooking Time: 40 minutes

Servings: 6

Ingredients:

1 red bell pepper, chopped

1 green bell pepper, chopped

1 tablespoon olive oil

2 yellow onions, chopped

6 garlic cloves, minced

24 ounces black-eyed peas, soaked overnight and drained

4 cups veggie stock

2 tablespoons chili powder, mild

2 teaspoons cumin, ground

½ teaspoon chipotle powder

2 teaspoons smoked paprika

30 ounces canned tomatoes, no-salt-added, chopped

2 cups corn

A pinch of black pepper

Directions:

Heat up a pot with the oil over medium heat, add the onions and the garlic, stir and cook for 5 minutes.

Add red and green bell pepper, chili powder, cumin, chipotle powder, smoked paprika and black pepper, stir and cook for 5 minutes more.

Add peas, stock, tomatoes and corn, stir, cover the pot and cook over medium heat for 30 minutes.

Divide into bowls and serve for lunch.

Nutrition:

Calories: 270

Protein: 12 G

Fat: 2 G

Carbs: 13 G

44.   Mediterranean Chicken

Preparation Time: 10 minutes

Cooking Time: 2 hours and 30 minutes

Servings: 4

Ingredients:

1 pound chicken breasts, skinless and boneless

2 tomatoes, chopped

1 cup low-sodium chicken stock

½ red bell pepper, chopped

1 yellow onion, sliced

Zest of 1 lemon, grated

Juice of 1 lemon

Black pepper to the taste

¾ cup whole wheat orzo

½ cup black olives, pitted

2 tablespoons scallions, chopped

Directions:

In your slow cooker, mix chicken with tomatoes, stock, bell pepper, onion, lemon zest, lemon juice and black pepper to the taste, cover and cook on High for 2 hours.

Add black olives and orzo, toss, cover, cook on high for 30 minutes more, divide everything between plates and serve with chopped scallions on top.

Nutrition: Calories: 211   Protein: 4 G

Fat: 3 G   Carbs: 12 G

45.   Grilled Eggplant Lunch Salad

Preparation Time: 10 minutes

Cooking Time: 20 minutes

Servings: 4

Ingredients:

1 tomato, diced

1 eggplant, pricked

A pinch of salt and black pepper

¼ teaspoon ground turmeric

1½ teaspoons red wine vinegar

½ teaspoon chopped oregano

3 tablespoons olive oil

2 garlic cloves, minced

3 tablespoons chopped parsley

2 tablespoons chopped capers

Directions:

Heat up your grill over medium-high heat, add eggplant, cook for 15 minutes, turning from time to time, scoop flesh, roughly chop and put in a bowl. Add salt, pepper to the taste, tomatoes, turmeric, garlic, vinegar, oregano, parsley, oil and capers, toss and serve.

Nutrition: Calories: 192 Protein: 7 G

Fat: 7 G Carbs: 12 G

46.   Eggplant and Avocado Lunch Mix

Preparation Time: 10 minutes

Cooking Time: 10 minutes

Servings: 4

Ingredients:

1 eggplant, sliced

1 red onion, sliced

2 teaspoons olive oil

1 avocado, pitted and chopped

1 teaspoon mustard

1 tablespoon red wine vinegar

1 tablespoon chopped oregano

1 teaspoon raw honey

A pinch of salt and black pepper

1 tablespoon chopped parsley

Zest of 1 lemon

Directions:

Brush the onion slices and eggplant slices with the olive oil, place them on the preheated kitchen grill, cook for 5 minutes on each side and let cool down. Cut the veggies into cubes, put in a salad bowl, add avocado and toss. In a bowl, mix vinegar with mustard, oregano, honey, olive oil, salt and pepper, whisk well and add to the salad. Toss together and sprinkle the lemon zest and the parsley on top and serve.

Nutrition: Calories: 212   Protein: 7 G

Fat: 7 G   Carbs: 12 G

47. Mediterranean Grilled Pork Chops

Preparation Time: 1 day

Cooking Time: 20 minutes

Servings: 6

Ingredients:

2 pork chops

¼ cup olive oil

2 yellow onions, sliced

2 garlic cloves, minced

2 teaspoons mustard

1 teaspoon sweet paprika

Salt and black pepper to taste

½ teaspoon oregano, dried

½ teaspoon thyme, dried

A pinch of cayenne pepper

Directions:

In a small bowl, mix oil with garlic, mustard, paprika, black pepper, oregano, thyme and cayenne and whisk well.

In a bowl, combine onions with meat and mustard mix, toss to coat, cover and keep in the fridge for 1 day. Place meat on preheated grill pan over medium high heat, season with salt and cook for 10 minutes on each side.

Meanwhile, heat a pan over medium heat, add marinated onions, stir and sauté for 4 minutes.

Divide pork chops on plates, add sautéed onions on top and serve.

Nutrition:

Calories: 284

Protein: 12 G

Fat: 4 G

Carbs: 7 G

Dinner recipes

48.   Mushroom And Cheese Soup

Preparation time: 10 minutes

Cooking time: 20 minutes

Servings: 2

Ingredients:

1 cup cremini mushrooms, chopped

1 cup Cheddar cheese, shredded

2 cups of water

½ teaspoon salt

1 teaspoon dried thyme

½ teaspoon dried oregano

1 tablespoon fresh parsley, chopped

1 tablespoon olive oil

1 bell pepper, chopped

Directions:

Pour olive oil in the pan.

Add mushrooms and bell pepper. Roast the vegetables for 5 minutes over the medium heat.

Then sprinkle them with salt, thyme, and dried oregano.

Add parsley and water. Stir the soup well.

Cook the soup for 10 minutes.

After this, blend the soup until it is smooth and simmer it for 5 minutes more.

Add cheese and stir until cheese is melted.

Ladle the cooked soup into the bowls. It is recommended to serve soup hot.

Nutrition:

Calories 320,

Fat 26,

Fiber 1.4,

Carbs 7.4,

Protein 15.7

49.   Parmesan Tomato Soap

Preparation time: 10 minutes

Cooking time: 20 minutes

Servings: 4

Ingredients:

½ cup tomatoes, chopped

1 tablespoon tomato paste

1 teaspoon garlic, diced

2 cups beef broth

1 teaspoon chili pepper

2 oz Parmesan, grated

1/3 cup fresh cilantro, chopped

2 potatoes, chopped

Directions:

Mix up together tomatoes and tomato paste and transfer the mixture in the pan.

Add garlic and beef broth.

Add chopped potatoes and chili pepper.

Boil the ingredients for 15 minutes or until potato is soft.

Then blend the mixture with the help of the hand blender or in the food processor.

Add chopped cilantro and simmer the soup for 5 minutes.

Ladle the cooked soup in the serving bowls and top every bowl with Parmesan generously.

Nutrition:

Calories 148,

Fat 3.9,

Fiber 3.1,

Carbs 19.8,

Protein 9.2

50.   Merjimek

Preparation time: 7 minutes

Cooking time: 40 minutes

Servings: 4

Ingredients:

1 cup red lentils

3 tablespoons sunflower oil

1 teaspoon pepper paste

½ teaspoon chili pepper

½ teaspoon chili flakes

½ teaspoon salt

1 teaspoon butter

½ teaspoon paprika

½ teaspoon ground black pepper

4 cups of water

1 green pepper, chopped

2 potatoes, finely chopped

Directions:

Put butter in the pan and melt it.

Add chopped pepper and potatoes and roast the vegetables for 5 minutes over the medium heat. Stir them occasionally.

After this, add water, lentils, ground black pepper, paprika, salt, chili flakes, chili pepper, pepper paste, and oil. Stir the ingredients with the help of the spoon.

Close the lid and cook soup for 35 minutes over the medium heat.

The cooked soup should have tender puree texture.

Nutrition: Calories 354, Fat 12.2, Fiber 18, Carbs 47.7, Protein 14.6

51.   Chicken Leek Soup

Preparation time: 10 minutes

Cooking time: 35 minutes

Servings: 4

Ingredients:

1 cup cabbage, shredded

6 oz leek, chopped

½ yellow onion, diced

1-pound chicken breast, skinless, boneless

1 tablespoon butter

1 teaspoon salt

½ teaspoon dried oregano

½ teaspoon dried thyme

1 tablespoon canola oil

4 cups of water

Directions:

Chop the chicken breast into the cubes and place in the pan.

Add butter and canola oil.

Cook the chicken for 5 minutes. Stir it from time to time.

After this, add yellow onion and chopped leek.

Add salt, dried oregano, and thyme. Mix up the ingredients well and saute for 5 minutes.

Then add water and cabbage.

Close the lid and cook soup over the medium heat for 25 minutes.

Nutrition:

Calories 222,

Fat 9.4,

Fiber 1.6,

Carbs 8.5,

Protein 25.1

52. Meatball Soup

Preparation time: 10 minutes

Cooking time: 30 minutes

Servings: 4

Ingredients: 1 cup ground beef

1 tablespoon semolina   ½ teaspoon salt

1 egg yolk

½ teaspoon ground black pepper

4 cups chicken stock   1 carrot, chopped

1 yellow onion, diced   1 tablespoon butter

½ teaspoon turmeric   ½ teaspoon garlic powder

Directions:

Toss butter in the skillet and heat it up until it is melted.

Add onion and cook it until light brown.

Meanwhile, pour chicken stock in the pan.

Add garlic powder and turmeric.

Bring the liquid to boil. Add chopped carrot and boil it for 10 minutes.

In the mixing bowl, mix up together ground beef, semolina, salt, egg yolk, and ground black pepper.

Make the small sized meatballs.

Put the meatballs in the chicken stock.

Add cooked onion.

Cook the soup for 15 minutes over the medium-low heat.

Nutrition: Calories 143, Fat 8.8,

Fiber 1.2, Carbs 7.5,

Protein 8.8

53.   Lemon Lamb Soup

Preparation time: 10 minutes

Cooking time: 50 minutes

Servings: 8

Ingredients:

1 ½-pound lamb bone in

4 eggs, beaten

2 cups lettuce, chopped

1 tablespoon chives, chopped

½ cup fresh dill, chopped

½ cup lemon juice

1 teaspoon salt

½ teaspoon white pepper

2 tablespoons avocado oil

5 cups of water

Directions:

Chop the lamb roughly and place in the pan.

Add avocado oil and roast the meat for 10 minutes over the medium heat. Stir it with the help of spatula from time to time.

Then sprinkle the meat with white pepper and salt. Add water and bring the mixture to boil.

In the mixing bowl, whisk together eggs and lemon juice.

Add a ½ cup of boiling water from the pan and whisk the egg mixture until smooth.

Add dill, chives, and lettuce in the soup. Stir well.

Cook the soup for 30 minutes over the medium-high heat.

Then add egg mixture and stir it fast to make the homogenous texture of the soup.

Cook it for 3 minutes more.

Nutrition:

Calories 360,

Fat 22.9,

Fiber 0.8,

Carbs 2.9,

Protein 33.6

54.   Eggplant Soup

Preparation time: 10 minutes

Cooking time: 30 minutes

Servings: 4

Ingredients:

½ cup tomatoes, chopped

2 eggplants, trimmed

¼ cup fresh parsley, chopped

¼ cup fresh cilantro, chopped

1 yellow onion, diced

½ teaspoon ground cumin

½ teaspoon cayenne pepper

1 celery stalk, chopped

1 tablespoon olive oil

1 teaspoon salt

1 garlic clove, peeled

1 teaspoon butter

4 cups chicken stock

Directions:

Peel eggplants and sprinkle them with olive oil and salt.

Preheat the oven to 360F.

Put the eggplants in the tray and transfer it in the preheated oven.

Bake the vegetables for 25 minutes.

Meanwhile, pour chicken stock in the pan.

Add chopped tomatoes, parsley, cilantro, ground cumin, cayenne pepper, celery stalk, and diced garlic clove.

Simmer the mixture for 5 minutes.

Meanwhile, heat up the butter in the skillet.

Add onion and roast it until translucent.

Add the onion in the boiled chicken stock mixture.

When the eggplants are cooked, transfer them in the food processor and blend until smooth.

After this, put the blended eggplants in the chicken stock mixture.

Blend the soup with the help of the hand blender until you get a creamy texture.

Simmer the soup for 5 minutes.

Nutrition: Calories 137, Fat 5.7, Fiber 10.9, Carbs 21.2, Protein 4.2

55.   Lasagna Rolls

Preparation time: 20 minutes

Cooking time: 30 minutes

Servings: 2

Ingredients:

2 zucchini, trimmed

1 cup Mozzarella, shredded

1 cup ground beef

½ teaspoon salt

½ teaspoon ground black pepper

½ teaspoon ground paprika

½ teaspoon dried oregano

¼ teaspoon cayenne pepper

1/3 cup tomato sauce

1teaspoon olive oil

¼ cup Cheddar cheese, shredded

1/3 cup chicken stock

Directions:

Slice the zucchini lengthwise.

In the mixing bowl, mix up together salt, ground beef, ground black pepper, ground paprika, and cayenne pepper.

Spread every zucchini slice with ground beef mixture and roll them.

Brush the casserole mold with olive oil from inside and arrange zucchini rolls.

Top every zucchini rolls with Mozzarella and Cheddar cheese.

Then mix up together tomato sauce, dried oregano, and chicken stock.

Pour the liquid over zucchini.

Cover the casserole mold with foil and secure the edges.

Bake lasagna rolls for 30 minutes at 355F.

Nutrition:
Calories 357,
Fat 23.7,
Fiber 3.3,
Carbs 11.4,
Protein 26.3

56.   Tortilla Wraps With Hummus

Preparation time: 10 minutes

Cooking time: 10 minutes

Servings: 2

Ingredients:

2 corn tortillas

1 cup Romaine lettuce, chopped

4 teaspoons hummus

1 tablespoon lemon juice

¼ teaspoon cayenne pepper

8 oz chicken fillet

½ teaspoon olive oil

½ teaspoon salt

Directions:

Slice the chicken fillet onto 2 fillets.

Rub every chicken fillet with cayenne pepper, olive oil, and salt.

Heat up the skillet well.

Place the chicken fillets in the skillet and roast them for 4 minutes from each side over the medium heat.

Meanwhile, spread one side of the corn tortillas with hummus.

Arrange the chopped lettuce on hummus and sprinkle with lemon juice.

Then add hot roasted chicken fillet and roll the tortillas (wrap). Secure every wrap with a toothpick.

Nutrition:

Calories 300,

Fat 11.3,

Fiber 2.3,

Carbs 13.2,

Protein 35.1

57.   Tomato & Chicken Skillet

Preparation time: 10 minutes

Cooking time: 20 minutes

Servings: 4

Ingredients:

1 cup tomatoes

1-pound chicken breast, skinless, boneless

3 bell peppers, chopped

½ cup of water

1 jalapeno pepper, chopped

½ teaspoon salt

1 tablespoon olive oil

Directions:

Chop tomatoes into the tiny pieces.

Then chop the chicken breast into the medium cubes.

Pour olive oil in the skillet and heat it up.

Add chicken breast cubes and roast them for 5 minutes.

After this, add chopped bell pepper and jalapeno pepper. Stir the ingredients well and cook for 5 minutes.

Add salt and tomatoes. Mix up well.

Cook the ingredients for 5 minutes and add water.

Stir it well.

Close the lid and cook the meal for 5 minutes more.

Nutrition:
Calories 197,
Fat 6.7,
Fiber 1.8,
Carbs 8.7,
Protein 25.4

58. Seafood Wraps With Avocado

Preparation time: 10 minutes

Cooking time: 6 minutes

Servings: 3

Ingredients:

3 corn tortillas

5 oz shrimps, peeled

3 oz crab meat, chopped

1 avocado, peeled, pitted

2 tablespoons Greek yogurt

¼ teaspoon minced garlic

½ teaspoon cayenne pepper

¾ teaspoon ground coriander

1 teaspoon butter

¼ cup heavy cream

1 cucumber, trimmed

Directions:

Pour heavy cream in the saucepan.

Add crab meat, shrimps, minced garlic, cayenne pepper, butter, and ground coriander.

Boil the seafood for 6 minutes.

After this, spread the tortillas with Greek yogurt from one side.

Cut avocado and cucumber into the wedges.

Arrange them on the tortillas.

Then add the seafood mixture.

Wrap the tortillas carefully and secure with the toothpicks.

Nutrition:
Calories 340,
Fat 20.4,
Fiber 6.6,
Carbs 22.3,
Protein 18.8

59. Carrot Soap

Preparation time: 10 minutes

Cooking time: 35 minutes

Servings: 6

Ingredients:

5 cups beef broth

4 carrots, peeled

1 teaspoon dried thyme

½ teaspoon ground cumin

1 teaspoon salt

1 ½ cup potatoes, chopped

1 tablespoon olive oil

½ teaspoon ground black pepper

1 tablespoon lemon juice

1/3 cup fresh parsley, chopped

1 chili pepper, chopped

1 tablespoon tomato paste

1 tablespoon sour cream

Directions:

Line the baking tray with baking paper.

Put sweet potatoes and carrot on the tray and sprinkle with olive oil and salt.

Bake the vegetables for 25 minutes at 365F.

Meanwhile, pour the beef broth in the pan and bring it to boil.

Add dried thyme, ground cumin, chopped chili pepper, and tomato paste.

When the vegetables are cooked, add them in the pan.

Boil the vegetables until they are soft.

Then blend the mixture with the help of the blender until smooth.

Simmer it for 2 minutes and add lemon juice. Stir well.

Then add sour cream and chopped parsley. Stir well.

Simmer the soup for 3 minutes more.

Nutrition:
Calories 123,
Fat 4.1,
Fiber 2.9,
Carbs 16.4,
Protein 5.3

60.   Wrapped Chopped Salad

Preparation time: 15 minutes

Servings: 4

Ingredients:

1 cup Monterey Jack cheese, shredded

1 avocado, chopped

½ cup radish, chopped

2 cups lettuce, teared

1 tomato, chopped

4 whole wheat tortillas

1 teaspoon olive oil

¼ teaspoon dried oregano

¼ teaspoon garlic powder

½ oz Plain yogurt

¼ teaspoon salt

Directions:

In the mixing bowl mix up together avocado, radish, lettuce, and tomato. Add cheese.

For the dressing: in the shallow bowl, whisk together salt, Plain yogurt, garlic powder, dried oregano, and olive oil.

Pour the dressing over the salad and give a good shake.

Then spoon the salad mixture down the center of every tortilla and wrap/roll them.

The cooked lunch should be served immediately; otherwise, it will not be crunchy.

Nutrition:

Calories 340,

Fat 20.7,

Fiber 7,

Carbs 28.9,

Protein 12.5

61. Chicken And Quinoa Salad With Pomegranate

Preparation time: 10 minutes

Cooking time: 20 minutes

Servings: 3

Ingredients:

½ cup quinoa

1 cup chicken stock

½ teaspoon salt

1 oz pomegranate seeds

8 oz chicken breast, skinless, boneless

1 tablespoon olive oil

1 cup lettuce, chopped

½ teaspoon paprika

½ teaspoon ground black pepper

1 teaspoon lemon juice

1 teaspoon butter

Directions:

In the pan combine together quinoa and chicken stock.

Add salt and boil the ingredients for 15 minutes or until quinoa will absorb all liquid.

Meanwhile, chop the chicken breast and sprinkle it with paprika and ground black pepper.

Place it in the skillet, add butter and roast for 10 minutes. Stir the chicken from time to time.

When the chicken and quinoa is cooked chill them to the room temperature and put in the salad bowl.

Add pomegranate seeds, lettuce, olive oil, and lemon juice.

Mix up the salad well.

Nutrition:

Calories 257,

Fat 9.8,

Fiber 2.4,

Carbs 21.1,

Protein 20.5

62.　Pasta E Fagioli Soap

Preparation time: 10 minutes

Cooking time:40 minutes

Servings: 6

Ingredients:

1 cup ditalini pasta, dried

6 cups of water

1 cup chicken stock

1 ½ cup ground beef

1 tablespoon olive oil

1 teaspoon salt

1 teaspoon ground black pepper

6 oz carrot, chopped

4 oz celery, chopped

3 tablespoons tomato sauce

1 tablespoon tomato paste

6 oz red kidney beans, canned, drained

1 teaspoon dried oregano

1 teaspoon dried basil

¼ teaspoon dried marjoram

6 teaspoons fresh parsley, chopped

1 teaspoon minced garlic

1 white onion, diced

Directions:

Pour olive oil in the skillet.

Add ground beef, salt, ground black pepper, and diced onion.

Cook the ingredients until they are cooked (appx.10 minutes over the medium heat).

Cook ditalini pasta according to the directions of the manufacturer.

Meanwhile, pour water and chicken stock in the pan.

Add carrot, celery, tomato sauce, tomato paste, and close the lid.

Bring the mixture to boil and simmer it for 10 minutes.

Then add cooked ground beef mixture.

Sprinkle it with dried oregano, basil, and marjoram.

Then add minced garlic and red kidney beans.

Close the lid and simmer the soup for 10 minutes over the medium heat.

After this, add chopped parsley and cooked pasta, and bring the soup to boil again.

Remove the cooked soup from the heat and close the lid.

Let the soup rest for at least 10 minutes before serving.

Nutrition:
Calories 278,
Fat 7.3,
Fiber 6.8,
Carbs 38.1,
Protein 16.3

63.   Mediterrannean Budha Bowl

Preparation time: 10 minutes

Cooking time: 25 minutes

Servings: 5

Ingredients:

1 cup chickpeas, canned, drained

½ teaspoon butter

½ teaspoon salt

½ teaspoon ground paprika

¾ teaspoon onion powder

6 oz quinoa, dried

12 oz chicken stock

2 tomatoes, chopped

1 cucumber, chopped

½ cup fresh spinach, chopped

½ cup arugula, chopped

½ cup lettuce chopped

1 tablespoon olive oil

4 teaspoons hummus

Directions:

Place chickpeas in the skillet. Add butter and salt.

Roast the chickpeas for 5 minutes over the high heat. Stir them from time to time.

After this, place quinoa and chicken stock in the pan.

Cook the quinoa for 15 minutes over the medium heat.

Then make the salad: mix up together tomatoes, cucumber, spinach, arugula, lettuce, and olive oil. Shake the salad gently.

Arrange roasted chickpeas in every serving bowl.

Add salad and hummus.

Then add quinoa. Buddha bowl is cooked.

Nutrition:
Calories 330,
Fat 8.4,
Fiber 10.9,
Carbs 51.6,
Protein 14.1

64.   Shrimp Crepes

Preparation time: 10 minutes

Cooking time: 10 minutes

Servings: 4

Ingredients:

4 eggs, beaten

4 teaspoons sour cream

1 cup shrimps, peeled, boiled

1 teaspoon butter

1 teaspoon olive oil

1/3 cup Mozzarella, shredded

½ teaspoon salt

1 teaspoon dried oregano

Directions:

In the mixing bowl, combine together sour cream, eggs, salt, and dried oregano.

Place butter and olive oil in the crepe skillet and heat the ingredients up.

Separate the egg liquid into 4 parts.

Ladle the first part of the egg liquid in the skillet and flatten it in the shape of crepe.

Sprinkle the egg crepe with ¼ part of shrimps and a small amount of Mozzarella.

Roast the crepe for 2 minutes from one side and then flip it onto another.

Cook the crepe for 30 seconds more.

Repeat the same steps with all remaining ingredients.

Nutrition:

Calories 148,

Fat 8.5,

Fiber 0.2,

Carbs 1.5,

Protein 16.1

65.   Carrot Noodles Salad

Preparation time: 15 minutes

Servings: 4

Ingredients:

2 carrots, peeled

1 tablespoon raisins, chopped

¼ cup walnuts, roughly chopped

5 oz Feta cheese, crumbled

3 teaspoons olive oil

3 teaspoon lemon juice

¼ teaspoon ground cardamom

¾ teaspoon saffron

¼ teaspoon sage

1 cup chickpeas, canned, drained

Directions:

Make the carrot noodles with the help of the spiralizer.

Place the carrot noodles in the salad bowl.

Add raisins, walnuts, and chickpeas. Shake the salad well.

Then make the dressing: mix up together sage, saffron, ground cardamom, lemon juice, and olive oil.

Pour the dressing over the salad.

Shake it well.

Sprinkle the cooked salad with crumbled Feta cheese and shake gently again.

Nutrition: Calories 375,
Fat 18.7, Fiber 10.2,
Carbs 37.6,
Protein 16.9

Dessert Recipes

66. Banana Shake Bowls

Preparation Time: 5 minutes

Cooking Time: 0 minutes

Servings: 4

Ingredients:

4 medium bananas, peeled

1 avocado, peeled, pitted and mashed

¾ cup almond milk

½ teaspoon vanilla extract

Directions:

In a blender, combine the bananas with the avocado and the other ingredients, pulse, divide into bowls and keep in the fridge until serving.

Nutrition: Calories 185 Fat 4.3

Fiber 4 Carbs 6 Protein 6.45

67. Cold Lemon Squares

Preparation Time: 30 minutes

Cooking Time: 0 minutes

Servings: 4

Ingredients: 1 cup avocado oil+ a drizzle

2 bananas, peeled and chopped

1 tablespoon honey   ¼ cup lemon juice

A pinch of lemon zest, grated

Directions:

In your food processor, mix the bananas with the rest of the ingredients, pulse well and spread on the bottom of a pan greased with a drizzle of oil.

Introduce in the fridge for 30 minutes, slice into squares and serve.

Nutrition: Calories 136 Fat 11.2 Fiber 0.2

Carbs 7 Protein 1.1

68.   Blackberry and Apples Cobbler

Preparation Time: 10 minutes

Cooking Time: 30 minutes

Servings: 6

Ingredients:

¾ cup stevia

6 cups blackberries

¼ cup apples, cored and cubed

¼ teaspoon baking powder

1 tablespoon lime juice

½ cup almond flour

½ cup water

3 and ½ tablespoon avocado oil

Cooking spray

Directions:

In a bowl, mix the berries with half of the stevia and lemon juice, sprinkle some flour all over, whisk and pour into a baking dish greased with cooking spray.

In another bowl, mix flour with the rest of the sugar, baking powder, the water and the oil, and stir the whole thing with your hands.

Spread over the berries, introduce in the oven at 375 degrees F and bake for 30 minutes. Serve warm.

Nutrition: Calories 221

Fat 6.3 Fiber 3.3 Carbs 6 Protein 9

69.   Black Tea Cake

Preparation Time: 10 minutes

Cooking Time: 35 minutes

Servings: 8

Ingredients:

6 tablespoons black tea powder

2 cups almond milk, warmed up

1 cup avocado oil

2 cups stevia

4 eggs

2 teaspoons vanilla extract

3 and ½ cups almond flour

1 teaspoon baking soda

3 teaspoons baking powder

Directions:

In a bowl, combine the almond milk with the oil, stevia and the rest of the ingredients and whisk well.

Pour this into a cake pan lined with parchment paper, introduce in the oven at 350 degrees F and bake for 35 minutes.

Leave the cake to cool down, slice and serve.

Nutrition: Calories 200 Fat 6.4

Fiber 4 Carbs 6.5 Protein 5.4

70.   Green Tea and Vanilla Cream

Preparation Time: 2 hours

Cooking Time: 0 minutes

Servings: 4

Ingredients:

14 ounces almond milk, hot

2 tablespoons green tea powder

14 ounces heavy cream

3 tablespoons stevia

1 teaspoon vanilla extract

1 teaspoon gelatin powder

Directions:

In a bowl, combine the almond milk with the green tea powder and the rest of the ingredients, whisk well, cool down, divide into cups and keep in the fridge for 2 hours before serving.

Nutrition:

Calories 120

Fat 3

Fiber 3

Carbs 7

Protein 4

71. Figs Pie

Preparation Time: 10 minutes

Cooking Time: 1 hour

Servings: 8

Ingredients:

½ cup stevia

6 figs, cut into quarters

½ teaspoon vanilla extract

1 cup almond flour

4 eggs, whisked

Directions:

Spread the figs on the bottom of a springform pan lined with parchment paper.

In a bowl, combine the other ingredients, whisk and pour over the figs,

Bake at 375 digress F for 1 hour, flip the pie upside down when it's done and serve.

Nutrition: Calories 200 Fat 4.4

Fiber 3

Carbs 7.6

Protein 8

72. Cherry Cream

Preparation Time: 2 hours

Cooking Time: 0 minutes

Servings: 4

Ingredients:

2 cups cherries, pitted and chopped

1 cup almond milk

½ cup whipping cream

3 eggs, whisked

1/3 cup stevia

1 teaspoon lemon juice

½ teaspoon vanilla extract

Directions:

In your food processor, combine the cherries with the milk and the rest of the ingredients, pulse well, divide into cups and keep in the fridge for 2 hours before serving.

Nutrition: Calories 200 Fat 4.5

Fiber 3.3   Carbs 5.6

Protein 3.4

73.   Strawberries Cream

Preparation Time: 10 minutes

Cooking Time: 20 minutes

Servings: 4

Ingredients:

½ cup stevia

2 pounds strawberries, chopped

1 cup almond milk

Zest of 1 lemon, grated

½ cup heavy cream

3 egg yolks, whisked

Directions:

Heat up a pan with the milk over medium-high heat, add the stevia and the rest of the ingredients, whisk well, simmer for 20 minutes, divide into cups and serve cold.

Nutrition: Calories 152 Fat 4.4

Fiber 5.5 Carbs 5.1

Protein 0.8

74.   Apples and Plum Cake

Preparation Time: 10 minutes

Cooking Time: 40 minutes

Servings: 4

Ingredients: 7 ounces almond flour

1 egg, whisked   5 tablespoons stevia

3 ounces warm almond milk

2 pounds plums, pitted and cut into quarters

2 apples, cored and chopped

Zest of 1 lemon, grated

1 teaspoon baking powder

Directions:

In a bowl, mix the almond milk with the egg, stevia, and the rest of the ingredients except the cooking spray and whisk well.

Grease a cake pan with the oil, pour the cake mix inside, introduce in the oven and bake at 350 degrees F for 40 minutes.

Cool down, slice and serve.

Nutrition: Calories 209 Fat 6.4 Fiber 6

Carbs 8 Protein 6.6

75.   Cinnamon Chickpeas Cookies

Preparation Time: 10 minutes

Cooking Time: 20 minutes

Servings: 12

Ingredients:

1 cup canned chickpeas, drained, rinsed and mashed

2 cups almond flour

1 teaspoon cinnamon powder

1 teaspoon baking powder

1 cup avocado oil

½ cup stevia

1 egg, whisked

2 teaspoons almond extract

1 cup raisins

1 cup coconut, unsweetened and shredded

Directions:

In a bowl, combine the chickpeas with the flour, cinnamon and the other ingredients, and whisk well until you obtain a dough.

Scoop tablespoons of dough on a baking sheet lined with parchment paper, introduce them in the oven at 350 degrees F and bake for 20 minutes.

Leave them to cool down for a few minutes and serve.

Nutrition: Calories 200   Fat 4.5 Fiber 3.4

Carbs 9.5 Protein 2.4

76.   Cocoa Brownies

Preparation Time: 10 minutes

Cooking Time: 20 minutes

Servings: 8

Ingredients:

30 ounces canned lentils, rinsed and drained

1 tablespoon honey

1 banana, peeled and chopped

½ teaspoon baking soda

4 tablespoons almond butter

2 tablespoons cocoa powder

Cooking spray

Directions:

In a food processor, combine the lentils with the honey and the other ingredients except the cooking spray and pulse well.

Pour this into a pan greased with cooking spray, spread evenly, introduce in the oven at 375 degrees F and bake for 20 minutes.

Cut the brownies and serve cold.

Nutrition: Calories 200 Fat 4.5 Fiber 2.4

Carbs 8.7 Protein 4.3

77.   Cardamom Almond Cream

Preparation Time: 30 minutes

Cooking Time: 0 minutes

Servings: 4

Ingredients:

Juice of 1 lime

½ cup stevia

1 and ½ cups water

3 cups almond milk

½ cup honey

2 teaspoons cardamom, ground

1 teaspoon rose water

1 teaspoon vanilla extract

Directions:

In a blender, combine the almond milk with the cardamom and the rest of the ingredients, pulse well, divide into cups and keep in the fridge for 30 minutes before serving.

Nutrition: Calories 283 Fat 11.8 Fiber 0.3

Carbs   Protein 7.1

78.   Banana Cinnamon Cupcakes

Preparation Time: 10 minutes

Cooking Time: 20 minutes

Servings: 4

Ingredients:

4 tablespoons avocado oil

4 eggs

½ cup orange juice

2 teaspoons cinnamon powder

1 teaspoon vanilla extract

2 bananas, peeled and chopped

¾ cup almond flour

½ teaspoon baking powder

Cooking spray

Directions:

In a bowl, combine the oil with the eggs, orange juice and the other ingredients except the cooking spray, whisk well, pour in a cupcake pan greased with the cooking spray, introduce in the oven at 350 degrees F and bake for 20 minutes.

Cool the cupcakes down and serve.

Nutrition: Calories 142 Fat 5.8

Fiber 4.2 Carbs 5.7 Protein 1.6

79.   Rhubarb and Apples Cream

Preparation Time: 10 minutes

Cooking Time: 0 minutes

Servings: 6

Ingredients:

3 cups rhubarb, chopped

1 and ½ cups stevia

2 eggs, whisked

½ teaspoon nutmeg, ground

1 tablespoon avocado oil

1/3 cup almond milk

Directions:

In a blender, combine the rhubarb with the stevia and the rest of the ingredients, pulse well, divide into cups and serve cold.

Nutrition: Calories 200 Fat 5.2 Fiber 3.4

Carbs 7.6 Protein 2.5

80.   Almond Rice Dessert

Preparation Time: 10 minutes

Cooking Time: 20 minutes

Servings: 4

Ingredients:

1 cup white rice

2 cups almond milk

1 cup almonds, chopped

½ cup stevia

1 tablespoon cinnamon powder

½ cup pomegranate seeds

Directions:

In a pot, mix the rice with the milk and stevia, bring to a simmer and cook for 20 minutes, stirring often.

Add the rest of the ingredients, stir, divide into bowls and serve.

Nutrition:

Calories 234 Fat 9.5 Fiber 3.4

Carbs 12.4 Protein 6.5

81.   Peach Sorbet

Preparation Time: 2 hours

Cooking Time: 10 minutes

Servings: 4

Ingredients:

2 cups apple juice

1 cup stevia

2 tablespoons lemon zest, grated

2 pounds peaches, pitted and quartered

Directions:

Heat up a pan over medium heat, add the apple juice and the rest of the ingredients, simmer for 10 minutes, transfer to a blender, pulse, divide into cups and keep in the freezer for 2 hours before serving.

Nutrition: Calories 182 Fat 5.4

Fiber 3.4 Carbs 12 Protein 5.4

82.   Cranberries and Pears Pie

Preparation Time: 10 minutes

Cooking Time: 40 minutes

Servings: 4

Ingredients:

2 cup cranberries

3 cups pears, cubed

A drizzle of olive oil

1 cup stevia

1/3 cup almond flour

1 cup rolled oats

¼ avocado oil

Directions:

In a bowl, mix the cranberries with the pears and the other ingredients except the olive oil and the oats, and stir well.

Grease a cake pan with the a drizzle of olive oil, pour the pears mix inside, sprinkle the oats all over and bake at 350 degrees F for 40 minutes.

Cool the mix down, and serve.

Nutrition:

Calories 172

Fat 3.4

Fiber 4.3

Carbs 11.5

Protein 4.5

83.   Lemon Cream

Preparation Time: 1 hour

Cooking Time: 10 minutes

Servings: 6

Ingredients:

2 eggs, whisked

1 and ¼ cup stevia

10 tablespoons avocado oil

1 cup heavy cream

Juice of 2 lemons

Zest of 2 lemons, grated

Directions:

In a pan, combine the cream with the lemon juice and the other ingredients, whisk well, cook for 10 minutes, divide into cups and keep in the fridge for 1 hour before serving.

Nutrition:

Calories 200

Fat 8.5

Fiber 4.5

Carbs 8.6

Protein 4.5

84. Blueberries Stew

Preparation Time: 10 minutes

Cooking Time: 10 minutes

Servings: 4

Ingredients:

2 cups blueberries

3 tablespoons stevia

1 and ½ cups pure apple juice

1 teaspoon vanilla extract

Directions:

In a pan, combine the blueberries with stevia and the other ingredients, bring to a simmer and cook over medium-low heat for 10 minutes.

Divide into cups and serve cold.

Nutrition:

Calories 192

Fat 5.4

Fiber 3.4

Carbs 9.4

Protein 4.5

85. Mandarin Cream

Preparation Time: 20 minutes

Cooking Time: 0 minutes

Servings: 8

Ingredients:

2 mandarins, peeled and cut into segments

Juice of 2 mandarins

2 tablespoons stevia

4 eggs, whisked

¾ cup stevia

¾ cup almonds, ground

Directions:

In a blender, combine the mandarins with the mandarins juice and the other ingredients, whisk well, divide into cups and keep in the fridge for 20 minutes before serving.

Nutrition: Calories 106 Fat 3.4

Fiber 0

Carbs 2.4

Protein 4

86.   Creamy Mint Strawberry Mix

Preparation Time: 10 minutes

Cooking Time: 30 minutes

Servings: 6

Ingredients:

Cooking spray

¼ cup stevia

1 and ½ cup almond flour

1 teaspoon baking powder

1 cup almond milk

1 egg, whisked

2 cups strawberries, sliced

1 tablespoon mint, chopped

1 teaspoon lime zest, grated

½ cup whipping cream

Directions:

In a bowl, combine the almond with the strawberries, mint and the other ingredients except the cooking spray and whisk well.

Grease 6 ramekins with the cooking spray, pour the strawberry mix inside, introduce in the oven and bake at 350 degrees F for 30 minutes.

Cool down and serve.

Nutrition:

Calories 200

Fat 6.3

Fiber 2

Carbs 6.5

Protein 8

87.   Vanilla Cake

Preparation Time: 10 minutes

Cooking Time: 25 minutes

Servings: 10

Ingredients:

3 cups almond flour

3 teaspoons baking powder

1 cup olive oil

1 and ½ cup almond milk

1 and 2/3 cup stevia

2 cups water

1 tablespoon lime juice

2 teaspoons vanilla extract

Cooking spray

Directions:

In a bowl, mix the almond flour with the baking powder, the oil and the rest of the ingredients except the cooking spray and whisk well.

Pour the mix into a cake pan greased with the cooking spray, introduce in the oven and bake at 370 degrees F for 25 minutes.

Leave the cake to cool down, cut and serve!

Nutrition:

Calories 200

Fat 7.6

Fiber 2.5

Carbs 5.5

Protein 4.5

88.   Pumpkin Cream

Preparation Time: 5 minutes

Cooking Time: 5 minutes

Servings: 2

Ingredients:

2 cups canned pumpkin flesh

2 tablespoons stevia

1 teaspoon vanilla extract

2 tablespoons water

A pinch of pumpkin spice

Directions:

In a pan, combine the pumpkin flesh with the other ingredients, simmer for 5 minutes, divide into cups and serve cold.

Nutrition:

Calories 192

Fat 3.4 Fiber 4.5

Carbs 7.6

Protein 3.5

89.   Chia and Berries Smoothie Bowl

Preparation Time: 5 minutes

Cooking Time: 0 minutes

Servings: 2

Ingredients:

1 and ½ cup almond milk

1 cup blackberries

¼ cup strawberries, chopped

1 and ½ tablespoons chia seeds

1 teaspoon cinnamon powder

Directions:

In a blender, combine the blackberries with the strawberries and the rest of the ingredients, pulse well, divide into small bowls and serve cold.

Nutrition: Calories 182 Fat 3.4

Fiber 3.4

Carbs 8.4

Protein 3

90.   Minty Coconut Cream

Preparation Time: 4 minutes

Cooking Time: 0 minutes

Servings: 2

Ingredients:

1 banana, peeled

2 cups coconut flesh, shredded

3 tablespoons mint, chopped

1 and ½ cups coconut water

2 tablespoons stevia

½ avocado, pitted and peeled

Directions:

In a blender, combine the coconut with the banana and the rest of the ingredients, pulse well, divide into cups and serve cold.

Nutrition:

Calories 193

Fat 5.4

Fiber 3.4 Carbs 7.6

Protein 3

91.   Watermelon Cream

Preparation Time: 15 minutes

Cooking Time: 0 minutes

Servings: 2

Ingredients:

1 pound watermelon, peeled and chopped

1 teaspoon vanilla extract

1 cup heavy cream

1 teaspoon lime juice

2 tablespoons stevia

Directions:

In a blender, combine the watermelon with the cream and the rest of the ingredients, pulse well, divide into cups and keep in the fridge for 15 minutes before serving.

Nutrition:

Calories 122

Fat 5.7

Fiber 3.2

Carbs 5.3

Protein 0.4

92.   Grapes Stew

Preparation Time: 10 minutes

Cooking Time: 10 minutes

Servings: 4

Ingredients:

2/3 cup stevia

1 tablespoon olive oil

1/3 cup coconut water

1 teaspoon vanilla extract

1 teaspoon lemon zest, grated

2 cup red grapes, halved

Directions:

Heat up a pan with the water over medium heat, add the oil, stevia and the rest of the ingredients, toss, simmer for 10 minutes, divide into cups and serve.

Nutrition:

Calories 122

Fat 3.7 Fiber 1.2

Carbs 2.3 Protein 0.4

93. Cocoa Sweet Cherry Cream

Preparation Time: 2 hours

Cooking Time: 0 minutes

Servings: 4

Ingredients:

½ cup cocoa powder

¾ cup red cherry jam

¼ cup stevia

2 cups water

1 pound cherries, pitted and halved

Directions:

In a blender, mix the cherries with the water and the rest of the ingredients, pulse well, divide into cups and keep in the fridge for 2 hours before serving.

Nutrition:

Calories 162

Fat 3.4 Fiber 2.4

Carbs 5

Protein 1

94. Apple Couscous Pudding

Preparation Time: 10 minutes

Cooking Time: 25 minutes

Servings: 4

Ingredients:

½ cup couscous

1 and ½ cups milk

¼ cup apple, cored and chopped

3 tablespoons stevia

½ teaspoon rose water

1 tablespoon orange zest, grated

Directions:

Heat up a pan with the milk over medium heat, add the couscous and the rest of the ingredients, whisk, simmer for 25 minutes, divide into bowls and serve.

Nutrition: Calories 150

Fat 4.5 Fiber 5.5

Carbs 7.5

Protein 4

95.   Ricotta Ramekins

Preparation Time: 10 minutes

Cooking Time: 1 hour

Servings: 4

Ingredients:

6 eggs, whisked

1 and ½ pounds ricotta cheese, soft

½ pound stevia

1 teaspoon vanilla extract

½ teaspoon baking powder

Cooking spray

Directions:

In a bowl, mix the eggs with the ricotta and the other ingredients except the cooking spray and whisk well.

Grease 4 ramekins with the cooking spray, pour the ricotta cream in each and bake at 360 degrees F for 1 hour.   Serve cold.

Nutrition: Calories 180

Fat 5.3 Fiber 5.4

Carbs 11.5 Protein 4

96.   Papaya Cream

Preparation Time: 10 minutes

Cooking Time: 0 minutes

Servings: 2

Ingredients:

1 cup papaya, peeled and chopped

1 cup heavy cream

1 tablespoon stevia

½ teaspoon vanilla extract

Directions:

In a blender, combine the cream with the papaya and the other ingredients, pulse well, divide into cups and serve cold.

Nutrition:

Calories 182

Fat 3.1

Fiber 2.3

Carbs 3.5

Protein 2

97.   Almonds and Oats Pudding

Preparation Time: 10 minutes

Cooking Time: 15 minutes

Servings: 4

Ingredients:

1 tablespoon lemon juice

Zest of 1 lime

1 and ½ cups almond milk

1 teaspoon almond extract

½ cup oats

2 tablespoons stevia

½ cup silver almonds, chopped

Directions:

In a pan, combine the almond milk with the lime zest and the other ingredients, whisk, bring to a simmer and cook over medium heat for 15 minutes.

Divide the mix into bowls and serve cold.

Nutrition: Calories 174 Fat 12.1

Fiber 3.2 Carbs 3.9

Protein 4.8

98.   Chocolate Cups

Preparation Time: 2 hours

Cooking Time: 0 minutes

Servings: 6

Ingredients:

½ cup avocado oil

1 cup, chocolate, melted

1 teaspoon matcha powder

3 tablespoons stevia

Directions:

In a bowl, mix the chocolate with the oil and the rest of the ingredients, whisk really well, divide into cups and keep in the freezer for 2 hours before serving.

Nutrition:

Calories 174

Fat 9.1

Fiber 2.2

Carbs 3.9

Protein 2.8

Salad Recipes

99. Sushi Appetizer

Preparation Time: 10 minutes

Servings:4

Ingredients:

1 large cucumber

3 tablespoons cream cheese

½ teaspoon chives

1 teaspoon lime juice

1 oz Feta cheese, crumbled

¼ teaspoon paprika

½ teaspoon ground black pepper

¾ teaspoon minced garlic

Directions:

Trim the ends of cucumber.

With the help of the vegetable slicer make the lengthwise slices from the cucumber.

Make the spread: churn together cream cheese, chopped chives, lime juice, crumbled Feta, paprika, ground black pepper, and minced garlic.

Then spread every cucumber slice with the cream cheese mixture.

Roll the cucumber slices and secure them with the help of the toothpick.

Nutrition:

calories 58,

Fat 4.2,

Fiber 0.5,

Carbs 3.7,

Protein 2.2

100.   Tuna Salad in Lettuce Cups

Preparation Time: 10 minutes

Cooking time: 10 minutes

Servings:6

Ingredients: 4 Romaine lettuce leaves

8 oz tuna fillet

1 teaspoon balsamic vinegar

½ teaspoon olive oil

1 tablespoon fresh dill, chopped

¼ teaspoon salt   ¾ teaspoon chili pepper

1 tomato, chopped   ¾ cup Plain yogurt

Directions: Rub the tuna fillet with salt and chili pepper.

Then drizzle the fish with olive oil.

Bake tuna for 10 minutes at 365F.

Then chill it little and chop.

In the bowl combine chopped tuna, Plain yogurt, tomato, fresh dill, and balsamic vinegar. Mix up well.

Fill the lettuce leaves with the tuna mixture.

Nutrition: Calories 152, Fat 11.2, Fiber 0.3, Carbs 3.4, Protein 9

101.   Rice Burgers

Preparation Time: 10 minutes

Cooking time: 30 minutes

Servings:4

Ingredients:

1/3 cup rice

1 cup of water

½ teaspoon salt

2 tablespoons ricotta cheese

1 egg

¼ cup yellow onion, diced

1 teaspoon sunflower oil

½ teaspoon ground black pepper

1 tablespoon wheat flour, whole grain

Directions:

Pour water in a pan. Add rice and salt.

Close the lid and boil rice for 15 minutes or until it will soak all liquid and will be done.

Meanwhile, heat up oil in the skillet.

Add diced onion and roast it until golden brown.

Combine cooked rice with onion.

Add ground black pepper, wheat flour, and egg.

Mix up the mixture. It should smooth but not liquid.

Then make medium size burgers.

Bake the burgers for 10 minutes at 355F.

Top the cooked appetizer with ricotta cheese.

Nutrition:Calories 104, Fat 3, Fiber 0.5, Carbs 15.1, Protein 3.7

102. Wheatberry Burgers

Preparation Time: 25 minutes

Cooking time: 15 minutes

Servings:6

Ingredients:

1 cup wheatberry, cooked

2 eggs

¼ cup ground chicken

1 tablespoon wheat flour, whole grain

1 teaspoon Italian seasoning

1 tablespoon olive oil

1 teaspoon salt

Directions:

In the mixing bowl mix up together wheatberry and ground chicken.

Crack eggs in the mixture.

Then add wheat flour, Italian seasoning, and salt.

Mix up the mass with the help of the spoon until homogenous.

Then make burgers and freeze them in the freezer for 20 minutes.

Heat up olive oil in the skillet.

Place frozen burgers in the hot oil and roast them for 4 minutes from each side over the high heat.

Then cook burgers for 10 minutes more over the medium heat. Flip them onto another side from time to time.

Nutrition: Calories 97, Fat 5.7,Fiber 1.5, Carbs 9.2, Protein 5.2

103. Tzatziki

Preparation Time: 10 minutes

Cooking time: 0 minutes

Servings:4

Ingredients:

1 large cucumber, trimmed

3 oz Greek yogurt

1 teaspoon olive oil

3 tablespoons fresh dill, chopped

1 tablespoon lime juice   ¾ teaspoon salt

1 garlic clove, minced

Directions:

Grate the cucumber and squeeze the juice from it.

Then place the squeezed cucumber in the bowl.

Add Greek yogurt, olive oil, dill, lime juice, salt, and minced garlic.

Mix up the mixture until homogenous.

Store tzatziki in the fridge up to 2 days.

Nutrition: Calories 44, Fat 1.8, Fiber 0.7, Carbs 5.1, Protein 3.2

104. Kale Wraps with Apple and Chicken

Preparation Time: 10 minutes

Cooking time: 10 minutes

Servings:4

Ingredients:

4 kale leaves

4 oz chicken fillet

½ apple

1 tablespoon butter

¼ teaspoon chili pepper

¾ teaspoon salt

1 tablespoon lemon juice

¾ teaspoon dried thyme

Directions:

Chop the chicken fillet into the small cubes.

Then mix up together chicken with chili pepper and salt.

Heat up butter in the skillet.

Add chicken cubes. Roast them for 4 minutes.

Meanwhile, chop the apple into small cubes and add it in the chicken.

Mix up well.

Sprinkle the ingredients with lemon juice and dried thyme.

Cook them for 5 minutes over the medium-high heat.

Fill the kale leaves with the hot chicken mixture and wrap.

Nutrition: Calories 106,Fat 5.1,Fiber 1.1, Carbs 6.3, Protein 9

2 tomatoes, sliced

Directions:

Cut every tortilla into 2 triangles.

Then mix up together cream cheese, ricotta cheese, minced garlic, and dill.

Spread 6 triangles with cream cheese mixture.

Then place sliced tomato on them and cover with remaining tortilla triangles.

Nutrition: Calories 71, Fat 1.6, Fiber 2.1, Carbs 12.8, Protein 2.3

105.   Tomato Finger Sandwich

Preparation Time: 10 minutes

Cooking time: 0 minutes

Servings:6

Ingredients:

6 corn tortillas

1 tablespoon cream cheese

1 tablespoon ricotta cheese

½ teaspoon minced garlic

1 tablespoon fresh dill, chopped

106.   Parsley Cheese Balls

Preparation Time: 10 minutes

Cooking time: 1 minute

Servings:6

Ingredients:

1/3 cup Cheddar cheese, shredded

1 tablespoon dried dill

1 egg, beaten

½ teaspoon salt

2 tablespoons coconut flakes

3 tablespoons sunflower oil

Directions:

Mix up together shredded cheese with dried dill, salt, and coconut flakes.

Then add egg and stir carefully until homogenous.

After this make small balls from the cheese mixture.

Heat up sunflower oil in the skillet.

Place cheese balls in the hot oil and roast them for 10 seconds from each side.

Dry the cooked cheese balls with the help of the paper towel.

Nutrition:
Calories 105,

Fat 10.4,

Fiber 0.2,

Carbs 0.7,

Protein 2.6

107. Layered Dip

Preparation Time: 10 minutes

Cooking time: 0 minutes

Servings:12

Ingredients: ½ cup hummus

8 tablespoons tzatziki 1 teaspoon olive oil

1 cup tomatoes, chopped

1 cup cucumbers, chopped

1 tablespoon lemon juice

1/3 cup fresh parsley, chopped

1 jalapeno pepper, chopped

Directions:In the mixing bowl mix up together fresh parsley, lemon juice, olive oil, cucumbers, tomatoes, and chopped jalapeno pepper.   Then make the layer of ½ part of tomato mixture in the casserole mold or glass mold.Top it with the layer of hummus.Then add remaining tomato mixture and flatten it well. Top it with tzatziki and flatten well. Store the dip in the fridge for up to 3 hours.

Nutrition: Calories 49, Fat 3.6, Fiber 1, Carbs 3.3, Protein 1.1

108. Grilled Tempeh Sticks

Preparation Time: 5 minutes

Cooking time: 8 minutes

Servings:6

Ingredients:

11 oz soy tempeh

1 teaspoon olive oil

½ teaspoon ground black pepper

¼ teaspoon garlic powder

Directions:

Cut soy tempeh into the sticks.

Sprinkle every tempeh stick with ground black pepper, garlic powder, and olive oil.

Preheat the grill to 375F.

Place the tempeh sticks in the grill and cook them for 4 minutes from each side. The time of cooking depends on the tempeh sticks size.

The cooked tempeh sticks will have a light brown color.

Nutrition: Calories 88,Fat 2.5, Fiber 3.6, Carbs 10.2, Protein 6.5

109. Sweet Potato Fries

Preparation Time: 10 minutes

Cooking time: 35 minutes

Servings:5

Ingredients:

1 teaspoon Zaatar spices

3 sweet potatoes

1 tablespoon dried dill

1 teaspoon salt

3 teaspoons sunflower oil

½ teaspoon paprika

Directions:

Pour water in the crockpot. Peel the sweet potatoes and cut them into the fries.

Line the baking tray with parchment.

Place the layer of the sweet potato in the tray.

Sprinkle the vegetables with dried dill, salt, and paprika.

Then sprinkle sweet potatoes with Zaatar and mix up well with the help of the fingertips.

Sprinkle the sweet potato fries with sunflower oil.

Preheat the oven to 375F.

Bake the sweet potato fries for 35 minutes. Stir the fries every 10 minutes.

Nutrition: Calories 28, Fat 2.9, Fiber 0.2, Carbs 0.6, Protein 0.2

110. Italian Style Potato Fries

Preparation Time: 10 minutes

Cooking time: 40 minutes

Servings:4

Ingredients:

1/3 cup baby red potatoes

1 tablespoon Italian seasoning

3 tablespoons canola oil

1 teaspoon turmeric

½ teaspoon of sea salt

½ teaspoon dried rosemary

1 tablespoon dried dill

Directions:

Cut the red potatoes into the wedges and transfer in the big bowl.

After this, sprinkle the vegetables with Italian seasoning, canola oil, turmeric, sea salt, dried rosemary, and dried dill.

Shake the potato wedges carefully.

Line the baking tray with baking paper.

Place the potatoes wedges in the tray. Flatten it well to make one layer.

Preheat the oven to 375F.

Place the tray with potatoes in the oven and bake for 40 minutes. Stir the potatoes with the help of the spatula from time to time.

The potato fries are cooked when they have crunchy edges.

Nutrition: Calories 122, Fat 11.6, Fiber 0.5, Carbs 4.5, Protein 0.6

101

111. Lemon Cauliflower Florets

Preparation Time: 15 minutes

Cooking time: 12 minutes

Servings:6

Ingredients:

1-pound cauliflower head, trimmed

3 tablespoons lemon juice

3 eggs, beaten

1 teaspoon salt

1 teaspoon ground black pepper

2 cups water, for cooking

3 tablespoons almond butter

1 teaspoon turmeric

Directions:

Place the cauliflower head in the pan.

Add water.

Boil the cauliflower for 8 minutes or until it is tender.

Then cool the vegetable well and separate it onto the florets.

Whisk together beaten eggs, salt, ground black pepper, and turmeric.

Dip every cauliflower floret in the egg mixture.

Toss the almond butter in the skillet and heat it up.

Roast the cauliflower florets for 2 minutes from each side over the medium heat.

When the cauliflower florets are golden brown, they are cooked.

Sprinkle the cooked florets with lemon juice.

Nutrition:

Calories 103,

Fat 6.9,

Fiber 2.9,

Carbs 6.3,

Protein 6.1

112.   Greek Style Nachos

Preparation Time: 7 minutes

Cooking time: 0 minutes

Servings:3

Ingredients:

3 oz tortilla chips

¼ cup Greek yogurt

1 tablespoon fresh parsley, chopped

¼ teaspoon minced garlic

2 kalamata olives, chopped

1 teaspoon paprika

¼ teaspoon ground thyme

Directions:

In the mixing bowl mix up together Greek yogurt, parsley, minced garlic, olives, paprika, and thyme.

Then add tortilla chips and mix up gently.

The snack should be served immediately.

Nutrition: Calories 81, Fat 1.6, Fiber 2.2, Carbs 14.1, Protein 3.5

113.   Cheesy Phyllo Bites

Preparation Time: 10 minutes

Cooking time: 15 minutes

Servings:8

Ingredients: 3 Phyllo sheets

½ cup Cheddar cheese   2 eggs, beaten

1 tablespoon butter

Directions:

Mix up together Cheddar cheese with eggs.

Spread the round springform pan with butter.

Place 2 Phyllo sheets inside the springform pan.

Place Cheddar cheese mixture over the Phyllo sheets and cover it with the remaining Phyllo dough sheet.

Preheat the oven to 365F.

Cut the Phyllo dough pie onto 8 pieces and bake for 15 minutes.

Nutrition: Calories 113,Fat 5.4, Fiber 0.4, Carbs 11.4, Protein 5

Mediterranean Diet Cookbook for Beginners

114. Cheddar Hot Pepper Dip

Preparation Time: 5 minutes

Cooking time: 10 minutes

Servings:6

Ingredients: 1 cup Cheddar cheese

¼ cup cilantro, chopped

1 chili pepper, chopped

1 teaspoon garlic powder   ¼ cup milk

Directions:

Bring the milk to boil.

Then add Cheddar cheese in the milk and simmer the mixture for 2 minutes. Stir it constantly.

After this, add cilantro, chili pepper, and garlic powder. Mix up the mixture well. If it doesn't get a smooth texture, use the hand blender to blend the mass.

It is recommended to serve the dip when it gets the room temperature.

Nutrition: Calories 83, Fat 6.5,Fiber 0.1, Carbs 1.2, Protein 5.1

115. Traditional Mediterranean Hummus

Preparation Time: 10 minutes

Cooking time: 45 minutes

Servings:7

Ingredients:

1 cup chickpeas, soaked

6 cups of water

½ cup lemon juice

3 tablespoon olive oil

1 teaspoon salt

1/3 teaspoon harissa

Directions:

Combine chickpeas and water and boil for 45 minutes or until chickpeas are tender.

Then transfer chickpeas in the food processor.

Add 1 cup of chickpeas water and lemon juice.

After this, add salt and harissa.

Blend the hummus until it is smooth and fluffy.

Add olive oil and pulse it for 10 seconds more.

Transfer the cooked hummus in the bowl and store it in the fridge up to 2 days.

Nutrition:

Calories 160,

Fat 7.9,

Fiber 5.

Carbs 17.8,

Protein 5.7

116.   Easy Nachos

Preparation Time: 10 minutes

Cooking time: 10 minutes

Servings:7

Ingredients:

1 cup nachos

1/3 cup Monterey Jack cheese, shredded

2 oz black olives, sliced

2 tomatoes, chopped

Directions:

Crash the nachos gently and arrange them in the casserole mold in one layer.

Make the layer of black olives and tomatoes over the nachos. Flatten the ingredients with the help of spatula if needed.

Then make the layer of cheese and cover casserole mold with foil. Secure the edges.

Bake the nachos for 10 minutes at 365F.

Then remove the foil from the mold and serve nachos in the casserole mold.

Nutrition:

Calories 133,

Fat 8,

Fiber 2.3,

Carbs 10.6,

Protein 5.4

117.   Salty Almonds

Preparation Time: 1 hour 10 minutes

Cooking time: 15 minutes

Servings:5

Ingredients:

1 cup almonds

3 tablespoons salt

2 cups of water

Directions:

Bring water to boil.

After this, add 2 tablespoons of salt in water and stir it.

When salt is dissolved, add almonds and let them soak for at least 1 hour.

Meanwhile, line the tray with baking paper and preheat oven to 350F.

Dry the soaked almonds with a paper towel well and arrange them in one layer in the tray.

Sprinkle buts with remaining salt.

Bake the snack for 15 minutes. Mix it from time to time with the help of the spatula or spoon.

Nutrition:
Calories 110,
Fat 9.5,
Fiber 2.4,
Carbs 4.1,
Protein 4

118. Zucchini Chips

Preparation Time: 15 minutes

Cooking time: 20 minutes

Servings:4

Ingredients: 1 zucchini

2 oz Parmesan, grated   ½ teaspoon paprika

1 teaspoon olive oil

Directions: Trim zucchini and slice it into the chips with the help of the vegetable slices.

Then mix up together Parmesan and paprika.

Sprinkle the zucchini chips with olive oil.

After this, dip every zucchini slice in the cheese mixture.

Place the zucchini chips in the lined baking tray and bake for 20 minutes at 375F.

Flip the zucchini sliced onto another side after 10 minutes of cooking.

Chill the cooked chips well.

Nutrition: Calories 64, Fat 4.3, Fiber 0.6, Carbs 2.3, Protein 5.2

119. Chili Chicken Wings

Preparation Time: 10 minutes

Cooking time: 20 minutes

Servings:3

Ingredients: 3 chicken wings, boneless

1 teaspoon chili pepper, minced

1tablespoon olive oil

1 teaspoon minced garlic

2 tablespoons balsamic vinegar

½ teaspoon salt

Directions: Make the chicken sauce: whisk together minced chili pepper, olive oil, minced garlic, balsamic vinegar, and salt.

 Preheat the oven to 360F.

 Line the baking tray with parchment.

 Rub the chicken wings with chicken sauce generously and transfer in the tray.

 Bake the poultry for 20 minutes. Flip them onto another side after 10 minutes of cooking.

Nutrition: Calories 138, Fat 11, Fiber 0.2, Carbs 3.8, Protein 5.9

120. Radish Flatbread Bites

Preparation Time: 10 minutes

Cooking time: 10 minutes

Servings:8

Ingredients:

2 tablespoons butter

1/3 cup milk

1 ½ cup wheat flour, whole grain

1 teaspoon salt

1 teaspoon avocado oil

1 cup radish

1 tablespoon cream cheese

Directions:

 Melt butter and combine it together with milk. Stir the liquid.

 Then mix up together flour with butter mixture.

 Knead the soft and non-sticky dough.

 Cut the dough into 8 pieces.

 Roll up every dough piece into the circle (flatbread).

Pour avocado oil in the skillet.

Roast the flatbreads for 1 minute from each side over the medium heat.

After this, slice the radish and mix it up with cream cheese and salt.

Top cooked flatbreads with radish.

Nutrition:

Calories 123,

Fat 3.8,

Fiber 0.9,

Carbs 18.9,

Protein 3

121.   Endive Bites

Preparation Time: 10 minutes

Cooking time: 0 minutes

Servings:10

Ingredients:

6 oz endive

2 pears, chopped

4 oz Blue cheese, crumbled

1 teaspoon olive oil

1 teaspoon lemon juice

¾ teaspoon ground cinnamon

Directions:

Separate endive into the spears (10 spears).

In the bowl combine chopped pears, olive oil, lemon juice, ground cinnamon, and Blue cheese.

Fill the endive spears with cheese mixture.

Nutrition:

Calories 72,

Fat 3.8,

Fiber 1.9,

Carbs 7.4,

Protein 2.8

122.   Eggplant Bites

Preparation Time: 15 minutes

Cooking time: 30 minutes

Servings:8

Ingredients:

2 eggs, beaten

3 oz Parmesan, grated

1 tablespoon coconut flakes

½ teaspoon ground paprika

1 teaspoon salt

2 eggplants, trimmed

Directions:

Slice the eggplants into the thin circles. Use the vegetable slicer for this step.

After this, sprinkle the vegetables with salt and mix up. Leave them for 5-10 minutes.

Then drain eggplant juice and sprinkle them with ground paprika.

Mix up together coconut flakes and Parmesan.

Dip every eggplant circle in the egg and then coat in Parmesan mixture.

Line the baking tray with parchment and place eggplants on it.

Bake the vegetables for 30 minutes at 360F. Flip the eggplants into another side after 12 minutes of cooking.

Nutrition: Calories 87, Fat 3.9, Fiber 5, Carbs 8.7, Protein 6.2

123.   Peanut Butter Yogurt Dip

Preparation Time: 10 minutes

Cooking time: 0 minutes

Servings:4

Ingredients:

2 tablespoons peanut butter

1 oz Greek Yogurt

1 teaspoon sesame seeds

½ teaspoon vanilla extract

1 tablespoon honey

Directions:

Put peanut butter and Greek yogurt in the big bowl.

With the help of the mixer mix up the mixture until fluffy.

After this, add sesame seeds, vanilla extract, and honey.

Stir it carefully.

Store the dip in the fridge.

Nutrition: Calories 74, Fat 4.5, Fiber 0.6, Carbs 6.5, Protein 2.9

124. Roasted Chickpeas

Preparation Time: 10 minutes

Cooking time: 3 hours

Servings:8

Ingredients:

1 cup chickpeas, canned

1 teaspoon salt

½ teaspoon ground coriander

½ teaspoon ground paprika

½ teaspoon dried thyme

¾ teaspoon cayenne pepper

2 tablespoons olive oil

Directions:

Drain the chickpeas and dry them carefully with the help of the towel.

After this, place them in the baking tray.

Mix up together salt, ground coriander, ground paprika, dried thyme, and cayenne pepper.

Sprinkle the chickpeas with spices and shake well.

After this, drizzle them with olive oil. Give a good shake again.

Preheat the oven to 375F.

Place the tray with chickpeas in the preheated oven and cook them for 35 minutes.

Flip the chickpeas on another side from time to time.

Nutrition:
Calories 122,
Fat 5.1,
Fiber 4.5,
Carbs 15.4,
Protein 4.9

125. Bell Pepper Muffins

Preparation Time: 15 minutes

Cooking time: 15 minutes

Servings:4

Ingredients:

4 eggs, beaten

4 teaspoons butter, softened

1 teaspoon baking powder

2 bell peppers, chopped

4 tablespoons wheat flour, whole grain

½ teaspoon ground black pepper

½ teaspoon salt

Directions:

Mix up together eggs, butter, baking powder, wheat flour, ground black pepper, and salt.

When the batter is smooth, add chopped bell pepper. Stir well.

Fill ½ part of every muffin mold with bell pepper batter.

Bake the muffins for 15 minutes at 365F.

Nutrition:
Calories 146,
Fat 8.4,
Fiber 1.1,
Carbs 11.6,
Protein 7

126.   Whole-Grain Lavash Chips

Preparation Time: 8 minutes

Cooking time: 10 minutes

Servings:4

Ingredients: 1 lavash sheet, whole grain

1 tablespoon canola oil   1 teaspoon paprika

½ teaspoon chili pepper   ½ teaspoon salt

Directions:

In the shallow bowl whisk together canola oil, paprika, chili pepper, and salt.

Then chop lavash sheet roughly (in the shape of chips).

Sprinkle lavash chips with oil mixture and arrange in the tray to get one thin layer.

Bake the lavash chips for 10 minutes at 365F. Flip them on another side from time to time to avoid burning.

Cool the cooked chips well.

Nutrition: Calories 73, Fat 4, Fiber 0.7, Carbs 8.4, Protein 1.6

127.   Quinoa Granola

Preparation Time: 10 minutes

Cooking time: 25 minutes

Servings:15

Ingredients:

1 cup rolled oats

6 oz quinoa

7 oz almonds, chopped

5 tablespoons maple syrup

3 tablespoons peanut butter

1 teaspoon ground cinnamon

1 tablespoon coconut flakes

Directions:

In the bog bowl mix up together rolled oats, quinoa, almonds, and coconut flakes.

Then add peanut butter and maple syrup.

Stir the mixture carefully with the help of the spoon.

Line the baking tray with parchment.

Transfer the quinoa mixture in the tray and flatten it well.

Bake granola for 25 minutes at 355F.

Chill the cooked granola well and crack on the servings.

Nutrition: Calories 177, Fat 9.4, Fiber 3.3, Carbs 19.1, Protein 5.9

128.   Cheesy Artichoke Dip

Preparation Time: 10 minutes

Cooking time: 10 minutes

Servings:6

Ingredients:

1 cup sour cream

1 cup fresh spinach

4 oz artichoke hearts, drained

1 cup Mozzarella cheese, shredded

1 teaspoon chili flakes

Directions:

Chop the artichoke hearts on the tiny pieces.

Put spinach in a blender and blend until smooth.

Mix up together spinach with artichokes. Add sour cream, Mozzarella cheese, and chili flakes. Stir well.

Transfer the mixture in the mold/pan and flatten it.

Bake the dip for 10 minutes at 360F.

Nutrition: Calories 105, Fat 8.9, Fiber 1.1,Carbs 4, Protein 3.3

Directions:

Place all ingredients in the food processor.

Blend the mixture until smooth.

After this, pour the cooked smoothie in the serving glass.

Nutrition: Calories 146, Fat 3.1, Fiber 2.7, Carbs 27.7, Protein 4.3

129.   Date and Fig Smoothie

Preparation Time: 5 minutes

Cooking time: 0 minutes

Servings:1

Ingredients:

1 date, pitted

1 fig, chopped

1 oz Greek yogurt

1/3 cup organic almond milk

1/3 teaspoon ground cardamom

1 teaspoon honey

130.   Cucumber Bites with Creamy Avocado

Preparation Time: 10 minutes

Cooking time: 0 minutes

Servings:5

Ingredients:

1 cucumber

5 cherry tomatoes

2 oz avocado, pitted

¼ teaspoon minced garlic

¼ teaspoon dried basil

¾ teaspoon sour cream

¾ teaspoon lemon juice

Directions:

Trim the cucumber and slice it on 5 thick slices.

After this, churn avocado until you get cream mass.

Add minced garlic, dried basil, sour cream, and lemon juice. Mix up well.

Spread the avocado mass over the cucumber slices and top it with cherry tomatoes.

Nutrition: Calories 56, Fat 2.7, Fiber 2.5, Carbs 8.1, Protein 1.7

131. Beetroot Chips

Preparation Time: 10 minutes

Cooking time: 15 minutes

Servings:4

Ingredients:

1 beetroot, peeled

1 teaspoon salt

1 tablespoon sunflower oil

Directions:

Thinly slice the beetroot and sprinkle with salt.

Add the sunflower oil and stir gently with the help of the spatula.

Arrange the beetroot chips in the tray one-by-one and bake for 12 minutes at 370F.

Then flip chips on another side and bake for 3 minutes more.

Nutrition:
Calories 42,
Fat 3.6,
Fiber 0.5,
Carbs 2.5,
Protein 0.4

Snack and appetizers

132. Meatballs Platter

Servings: 4

Preparation time: 10 minutes

Cooking time: 15 minutes

Ingredients: 1 pound beef meat, ground

¼ cup panko breadcrumbs

A pinch of salt and black pepper

3 tablespoons red onion, grated

¼ cup parsley, chopped

2 garlic cloves, minced

2 tablespoons lemon juice

Zest of 1 lemon, grated

1 egg

½ teaspoon cumin, ground

½ teaspoon coriander, ground

¼ teaspoon cinnamon powder

2 ounces feta cheese, crumbled

Directions: In a bowl, mix the beef with the breadcrumbs, salt, pepper and the rest of the ingredients except the cooking spray, stir well and shape medium balls out of this mix.

Arrange the meatballs on a baking sheet lined with parchment paper, grease them with cooking spray and bake at 450°F for 15 minutes.

Arrange the meatballs on a platter and serve as an appetizer.

Nutrition: Calories 300; Fat 15.4 g; Fiber 6.4 g, Carbs 22.4 g; Protein 35 g

133. Yogurt Dip

Servings: 6

Preparation time: 10 minutes

Cooking time: 0 minutes

Ingredients: 2 cups Greek yogurt

2 tablespoons pistachios, toasted and chopped

A pinch of salt and white pepper

2 tablespoons mint, chopped

1 tablespoon kalamata olives, pitted and chopped

¼ cup za'atar spice

¼ cup pomegranate seeds

1/3 cup olive oil

Directions: In a bowl, combine the yogurt with the pistachios and the rest of the ingredients, whisk well, divide into small cups and serve with pita chips on the side.

Nutrition: Calories 294; Fat 18 g; Fiber 1 g; Carbs 21 g; Protein 10 g

134. Tomato Bruschetta

Servings: 6

Preparation time: 10 minutes

Cooking time: 10 minutes

Ingredients: 1 baguette, sliced

1/3 cup basil, chopped

6 tomatoes, cubed

2 garlic cloves, minced

A pinch of salt and black pepper

1 teaspoon olive oil

1 tablespoon balsamic vinegar

½ teaspoon garlic powder

Cooking spray

Directions: Arrange the baguette slices on a baking sheet lined with parchment paper, grease them with cooking spray and bake at 400° F for 10 minutes.

In a bowl, mix the tomatoes with the basil and the remaining ingredients, toss well and leave aside for 10 minutes.

Divide the tomato mix on each baguette slice, arrange them all on a platter and serve.

Nutrition: Calories 162; Fat 4 g; Fiber 7 g; Carbs 29 g; Protein 4 g

135.   Artichoke Flatbread

Servings: 4

Preparation time: 10 minutes

Cooking time: 15 minutes

Ingredients: 5 tablespoons olive oil

2 garlic cloves, minced

2 tablespoons parsley, chopped

2 round whole wheat flatbreads

4 tablespoons parmesan, grated

½ cup mozzarella cheese, grated

14 ounces canned artichokes, drained and quartered

1 cup baby spinach, chopped

½ cup cherry tomatoes, halved

½ teaspoon basil, dried

Salt and black pepper to the taste

Directions: In a bowl, mix the parsley with the garlic and 4 tablespoons oil, whisk well and spread this over the flatbreads.

Sprinkle the mozzarella and half of the parmesan.

In a bowl, mix the artichokes with the spinach, tomatoes, basil, salt, pepper and the rest of the oil, toss and divide over the flatbreads as well.

Sprinkle the rest of the parmesan on top, arrange the flatbreads on a baking sheet lined with parchment paper and bake at 425° F for 15 minutes.

Serve as an appetizer.

Nutrition: Calories 223; Fat 11.2 g; Fiber 5.34 g, Carbs 15.5 g; Protein 7.4 g

136.   Red Pepper Tapenade

Servings: 4

Preparation time: 10 minutes

Cooking time: 0 minutes

Ingredients: 7 ounces roasted red peppers, chopped

½ cup parmesan, grated

1/3 cup parsley, chopped

14 ounces canned artichokes, drained and chopped

3 tablespoons olive oil

¼ cup capers, drained

1 and ½ tablespoons lemon juice

2 garlic cloves, minced

Directions: In your blender, combine the red peppers with the parmesan and the rest of the ingredients and pulse well.

Divide into cups and serve as a snack.

Nutrition: Calories 200; Fat 5.6 g; Fiber 4.5 g; Carbs 12.4 g; Protein 4.6 g

137. Coriander Falafel

Servings: 8

Preparation time: 10 minutes

Cooking time: 10 minutes

Ingredients: 1 cup canned garbanzo beans, drained and rinsed

1 bunch parsley leaves

1 yellow onion, chopped

5 garlic cloves, minced

1 teaspoon coriander, ground

A pinch of salt and black pepper

¼ teaspoon cayenne pepper

¼ teaspoon baking soda

¼ teaspoon cumin powder

1 teaspoon lemon juice

3 tablespoons tapioca flour

Olive oil for frying

Directions: In your food processor, combine the beans with the parsley, onion and the rest the ingredients except the oil and the flour and pulse well.

Transfer the mix to a bowl, add the flour, stir well, shape 16 balls out of this mix and flatten them a bit.

Heat up a pan with some oil over medium-high heat, add the falafels, cook them for 5 minutes on each side, transfer to paper towels, drain excess grease, arrange them on a platter and serve as an appetizer.

Nutrition: Calories 112; Fat 6.2 g; Fiber 2 g; Carbs 12.3 g; Protein 3.1g

138. Red Pepper Hummus

Servings: 6

Preparation time: 10 minutes

Cooking time: 0 minutes

Ingredients: 6 ounces roasted red peppers, peeled and chopped

16 ounces canned chickpeas, drained and rinsed

¼ cup Greek yogurt

3 tablespoons tahini paste

Juice of 1 lemon

3 garlic cloves, minced 1 tablespoon olive oil

A pinch of salt and black pepper

1 tablespoon parsley, chopped

Directions: In your food processor, combine the red peppers with the rest of the ingredients except the oil and the parsley and pulse well.

Add the oil, pulse again, divide into cups, sprinkle the parsley on top and serve as a party spread.

Nutrition: Calories 255; Fat 11.4 g; Fiber 4.5 g; Carbs 17.4 g; Protein 6.5 g

139. White Bean Dip

Servings: 4

Preparation time: 10 minutes

Cooking time: 0 minute

Ingredients: 15 ounces canned white beans, drained and rinsed

6 ounces canned artichoke hearts, drained and quartered

4 garlic cloves, minced

1 tablespoon basil, chopped

2 tablespoons olive oil

Juice of ½ lemon

Zest of ½ lemon, grated

Salt and black pepper to the taste

Directions: In your food processor, combine the beans with the artichokes and the rest of the ingredients except the oil and pulse well.

Add the oil gradually, pulse the mix again, divide into cups and serve as a party dip.

Nutrition: Calories 274; Fat 11.7 g; Fiber 6.5 g; Carbs 18.5 g; Protein 16.5 g

Hummus with Ground Lamb

Servings: 8

Preparation time: 10 minutes

Cooking time: 15 minute

Ingredients: 10 ounces hummus

12 ounces lamb meat, ground

½ cup pomegranate seeds

¼ cup parsley, chopped

1 tablespoon olive oil

Pita chips for serving

Directions: Heat up a pan with the oil over medium-high heat, add the meat, and brown for 15 minutes stirring often.

Spread the hummus on a platter, spread the ground lamb all over, also spread the pomegranate seeds and the parsley and serve with pita chips as a snack.

Nutrition: Calories 133; Fat 9.7 g; Fiber 1.7 g; Carbs 6.4 g; Protein 5

140.   Eggplant Dip

Servings: 4

Preparation time: 10 minutes

Cooking time: 40 minutes

Ingredients: 1 eggplant, poked with a fork

2 tablespoons tahini paste

2 tablespoons lemon juice

2 garlic cloves, minced

1 tablespoon olive oil

Salt and black pepper to the taste

1 tablespoon parsley, chopped

Directions: Put the eggplant in a roasting pan, bake at 400° F for 40 minutes, cool down, peel and transfer to your food processor.

Add the rest of the ingredients except the parsley, pulse well, divide into small bowls and serve as an appetizer with the parsley sprinkled on top.

Nutrition: Calories 121; Fat 4.3 g; Fiber 1 g; Carbs 1.4 g; Protein 4.3 g

141. Veggie Fritters

Servings: 8

Preparation time: 10 minutes

Cooking time: 10 minutes

Ingredients: 2 garlic cloves, minced

2 yellow onions, chopped

4 scallions, chopped

2 carrots, grated

2 teaspoons cumin, ground

½ teaspoon turmeric powder

Salt and black pepper to the taste

¼ teaspoon coriander, ground

2 tablespoons parsley, chopped

¼ teaspoon lemon juice

½ cup almond flour

2 beets, peeled and grated

2 eggs, whisked

¼ cup tapioca flour

3 tablespoons olive oil

Directions: In a bowl, combine the garlic with the onions, scallions and the rest of the ingredients except the oil, stir well and shape medium fritters out of this mix.

Heat up a pan with the oil over medium-high heat, add the fritters, cook for 5 minutes on each side, arrange on a platter and serve.

Nutrition: Calories 209; Fat 11.2 g; Fiber 3 g; Carbs 4.4 g; Protein 4.8 g

142. Bulgur Lamb Meatballs

Servings: 6

Preparation time: 10 minutes

Cooking time: 15 minute

Ingredients: 1 and ½ cups Greek yogurt

½ teaspoon cumin, ground

1 cup cucumber, shredded

½ teaspoon garlic, minced

A pinch of salt and black pepper

1 cup bulgur

2 cups water

1 pound lamb, ground

¼ cup parsley, chopped

¼ cup shallots, chopped

½ teaspoon allspice, ground

½ teaspoon cinnamon powder

1 tablespoon olive oil

Directions: In a bowl, combine the bulgur with the water, cover the bowl, leave aside for 10 minutes, drain and transfer to a bowl.

Add the meat, the yogurt and the rest of the ingredients except the oil, stir well and shape medium meatballs out of this mix.

Heat up a pan with the oil over medium-high heat, add the meatballs, cook them for 7 minutes on each side, arrange them all on a platter and serve as an appetizer.

Nutrition: Calories 300; Fat 9.6 g; Fiber 4.6 g; Carbs 22.6 g; Protein 6.6 g

143.   Cucumber Bites

Servings: 12

Preparation time: 10 minutes

Cooking time: 0 minutes

Ingredients: 1 English cucumber, sliced into 32 rounds

10 ounces hummus

16 cherry tomatoes, halved

1 tablespoon parsley, chopped

1 ounce feta cheese, crumbled

Directions: Spread the hummus on each cucumber round, divide the tomato halves on each, sprinkle the cheese and parsley on to and serve as an appetizer.

Nutrition: Calories 162; Fat 3.4 g; Fiber 2 g; Carbs 6.4 g; Protein 2.4 g

144.   Stuffed Avocado

Servings: 2

Preparation time: 10 minutes

Cooking time: 0 minute

Ingredients: 1 avocado, halved and pitted

10 ounces canned tuna, drained

2 tablespoons sun-dried tomatoes, chopped

1 and ½ tablespoon basil pesto

2 tablespoons black olives, pitted and chopped

Salt and black pepper to the taste

2 teaspoons pine nuts, toasted and chopped

1 tablespoon basil, chopped

Directions: In a bowl, combine the tuna with the sun-dried tomatoes and the rest of the ingredients except the avocado and stir.

Stuff the avocado halves with the tuna mix and serve as an appetizer.

Nutrition: Calories 233; Fat 9 g; Fiber 3.5 g; Carbs 11.4 g; Protein 5.6 g

145.   Wrapped Plums

Servings: 8

Preparation time: 5 minutes

Cooking time: 0 minutes

Ingredients: 2 ounces prosciutto, cut into 16 pieces

4 plums, quartered

1 tablespoon chives, chopped

A pinch of red pepper flakes, crushed

Directions: Wrap each plum quarter in a prosciutto slice, arrange them all on a platter, sprinkle the chives and pepper flakes all over and serve.

Nutrition: Calories 30; Fat 1 g; Fiber 0 g; Carbs 4 g; Protein 2 g

Cucumber Sandwich Bites

Servings: 12

Preparation time: 5 minutes

Cooking time: 0 minutes

Ingredients: 1 cucumber, sliced

8 slices whole wheat bread

2 tablespoons cream cheese, soft

1 tablespoon chives, chopped

¼ cup avocado, peeled, pitted and mashed

1 teaspoon mustard

Salt and black pepper to the taste

Directions: Spread the mashed avocado on each bread slice, also spread the rest of the ingredients except the cucumber slices. Divide the cucumber slices on the bread slices, cut each slice in thirds, arrange on a platter and serve as an appetizer.

Nutrition: Calories 187; Fat 12.4 g; Fiber 2.1 g; Carbs 4.5 g; Protein 8.2 g

146.   Cucumber Rolls

Servings: 6

Preparation time: 5 minutes

Cooking time: 0 minutes

Ingredients: 1 big cucumber, sliced lengthwise

1 tablespoon parsley, chopped

8 ounces canned tuna, drained and mashed

Salt and black pepper to the taste

1 teaspoon lime juice

Directions: Arrange cucumber slices on a working surface, divide the rest of the ingredients, and roll.

Arrange all the rolls on a platter and serve as an appetizer.

Nutrition:Calories 200; Fat 6 g; Fiber 3.4 g; Carbs 7.6 g;Protein 3.5 g

147.   Olives and Cheese Stuffed Tomatoes

Servings: 24

Preparation time: 10 minutes

Cooking time: 0 minutes

Ingredients: 24 cherry tomatoes, top cut off and insides scooped out

2 tablespoons olive oil

¼ teaspoon red pepper flakes

½ cup feta cheese, crumbled

2 tablespoons black olive paste

¼ cup mint, torn

Directions: In a bowl, mix the olives paste with the rest of the ingredients except the cherry tomatoes and whisk well. Stuff the cherry tomatoes with this mix, arrange them all on a platter and serve as an appetizer.

Nutrition: Calories 136; Fat 8.6 g;Fiber 4.8 g; Carbs 5.6 g; Protein 5.1 g

148.   Tomato Salsa

Servings: 6

Preparation time: 5 minutes

Cooking time: 0 minutes

Ingredients: 1 garlic clove, minced

4 tablespoons olive oil

5 tomatoes, cubed

1 tablespoon balsamic vinegar

¼ cup basil, chopped

1 tablespoon parsley, chopped

1 tablespoon chives, chopped

Salt and black pepper to the taste

Pita chips for serving

Directions: In a bowl, mix the tomatoes with the garlic and the rest of the ingredients except the pita chips, stir, divide into small cups and serve with the pita chips on the side.

Nutrition: Calories 160; Fat 13.7 g; Fiber 5.5 g; Carbs 10.1 g; Protein 2.2

149.   Chili Mango and Watermelon Salsa

Servings: 12

Preparation time: 5 minutes

Cooking time: 0 minutes

Ingredients: 1 red tomato, chopped

Salt and black pepper to the taste

1 cup watermelon, seedless, peeled and cubed

1 red onion, chopped

2 mangos, peeled and chopped

2 chili peppers, chopped

¼ cup cilantro, chopped

3 tablespoons lime juice

Pita chips for serving

Directions: In a bowl, mix the tomato with the watermelon, the onion and the rest of the ingredients except the pita chips and toss well. Divide the mix into small cups and serve with pita chips on the side.

Nutrition: Calories 62; Fat g; Fiber 1.3 g; Carbs 3.9 g; Protein 2.3 g

150.   Creamy Spinach and Shallots Dip

Servings: 4

Preparation time: 10 minutes

Cooking time: 0 minutes

Ingredients: 1 pound spinach, roughly chopped

2 shallots, chopped

2 tablespoons mint, chopped

¾ cup cream cheese, soft

Salt and black pepper to the taste

Directions: In a blender, combine the spinach with the shallots and the rest of the ingredients, and pulse well. Divide into small bowls and serve as a party dip.

Nutrition: Calories 204; Fat 11.5 g; Fiber 3.1 g; Carbs 4.2 g; rotein 5.9 g

151.   Feta Artichoke Dip

Servings: 8

Preparation time: 10 minutes

Cooking time: 30 minutes

Ingredients: 8 ounces artichoke hearts, drained and quartered

¾ cup basil, chopped

¾ cup green olives, pitted and chopped

1 cup parmesan cheese, grated

5 ounces feta cheese, crumbled

Directions: In your food processor, mix the artichokes with the basil and the rest of the ingredients, pulse well, and transfer to a baking dish.

Introduce in the oven, bake at 375° F for 30 minutes and serve as a party dip.

Nutrition: Calories 186; Fat 12.4 g; Fiber 0.9 g; Carbs 2.6 g; Protein 1.5 g

152.   Avocado Dip

Servings: 8

Preparation time: 5 minutes

Cooking time: 0 minutes

Ingredients: ½ cup heavy cream

1 green chili pepper, chopped

Salt and pepper to the taste

4 avocados, pitted, peeled and chopped

1 cup cilantro, chopped

¼ cup lime juice

Directions: In a blender, combine the cream with the avocados and the rest of the ingredients and pulse well. Divide the mix into bowls and serve cold as a party dip.

Nutrition: Calories 200; Fat 14.5 g; Fiber 3.8 g; Carbs 8.1 g; Protein 7.6 g

153. Goat Cheese and Chives Spread

Servings: 4

Preparation time: 10 minutes

Cooking time: 0 minutes

Ingredients: 2 ounces goat cheese, crumbled

¾ cup sour cream

2 tablespoons chives, chopped

1 tablespoon lemon juice

Salt and black pepper to the taste

2 tablespoons extra virgin olive oil

Directions: In a bowl, mix the goat cheese with the cream and the rest of the ingredients and whisk really well. Keep in the fridge for 10 minutes and serve as a party spread.

Nutrition: Calories 220; Fat 11.5 g; Fiber 4.8 g; Carbs 8.9 g; Protein 5.6 g

How to Implement the Mediterranean Diet into Your Lifestyle

We are all involved in being lean, losing weight, getting a good diet plan, getting rid of cardiovascular and health-related illnesses. Typically, once you have a good diet plan such as the Mediterranean diet pan, the chances are that you will eventually reduce the number of calories in your body resulting in decreased heart-related issues.

The other benefits include weight shedding,Fat burning and gradually slimming down. It is truly easy to implement diet plans like the Mediterranean diet plan. That's because you can't eat the gunk and bland vegetables that many people have to submit to just because they want to live longer and healthier.

You will enjoy delicious meals with the Mediterranean diet plan while still rising the chances of getting heart-related problems. Here are a few tips to help adopt the Mediterranean diet.

1. Decide on What Diet Type

Most of the people tend to worry about their diet plans consistently. They worry if it will work if they lose weight if they can reduce their chances of dying younger as a result of heart disease and cancer and, most importantly, worry if they can keep up with their diets. Okay, the thing is, if you really want to do this, you have to choose which choice you think works best for you.

There are two main dietary forms or regimens. You can do the form planned or the style Do-It-Yourself. It all depends on the makeup you have. For instance, some people don't like strict time tables and are more likely to fail to use them because they are instinctively opposed to things that make them feel like they're boxed in.

Though, other people find it exciting to chart a strategy and are more likely to stick to it. It all depends on the person that you are. So, whatever happens, just pick one out. If you don't know which group you're moving for, just go for one. You can always turn to the other, if you don't like it.

2. Find Recipes that Will Work for You

The taste of the people in the food is different. You need to find and stick to that which works for you. The basic components of the Mediterranean diet plan include, among others, olive oil, legumes, vegetables, nuts, grains, unprocessed carbohydrates, fish, reduced red meat consumption and saturated Fat.

Now, if you just like eating them like that, then it's all right. But if you want to make it much more fun, you'd have to find recipes that work. The South Beach Diet recipes, for example, are great and fun to cook. So, find recipes that inculcate these and which are based on the Mediterranean diet.

3. Get Creative With the Diet

Since following a few diet plans, the reason many people return to eating junk is that the diets are either dull, repetitive or lacking in flavor. So, what you should do is just go for those delicious meals. Get yourself creative with the recipes. Try something new, and something different. Chances are if you're looking well enough, you'll find lots of Mediterranean diet recipes that will last you for a whole year and more.

4. Be Disciplined

Because the Mediterranean diet is really simple to use and apply, it is hardly called a diet by some. I just see it as an alternative lifestyle and food choices that help you stay healthy and live longer. The secret, then, is discipline. Stay focused and who knows, you could just give yourself an extra 15 years of health and life.

Reasons Why a Mediterranean Diet in the 21st Century Is A Healthy Choice

With the vast number of diet plans, services, supplements and aids on the market, a diet plan that can and will better meet your needs now and into the future may seem almost impossible to choose. Most significantly, it can be difficult to discern whether one or the other of these different diet plans are actually a healthy path to follow. In many cases, fad diets are not really focused on the foundations of a healthy life.

When you decide what sort of diet plan or a diet plan or diet will best serve your needs and enhance your health in the future, you will want to look at the benefits that the Mediterranean diet can offer.

While there are multiple reasons why a balanced alternative is a Mediterranean diet, there are five main reasons why a good choice is a Mediterranean diet.

1.   The benefits of fruits, vegetables, Fiber and whole grains

Regular consumption of fresh fruit and vegetables is an important component of the Mediterranean diet. Medical experts and nutritionists generally agree that a person should eat around 5-6 servings of fresh fruit and vegetables (or steamed items) daily.

People who generally adhere to the Mediterranean diet eventually eat more than the minimum recommended amount of fruit and vegetables. As a result, nutritionists in different parts of the world have prescribed a Mediterranean-based program for its customers. Today doctors who recommend healthy eating habits to their patients often stick to the Mediterranean diet.

The Mediterranean diet contains healthy amounts of dietary Fiber and whole grains, in addition to fruit and vegetables. Fiber and whole grains have proven effective in reducing heart disease incidence and certain types of cancer.

The vast majority of the Fat a person consumes on the Mediterranean diet comes from olive oil. The Fat present in the Mediterranean diet is not, in other words, the unhealthy saturated Fat that can cause disease, obesity and other health concerns. Nonetheless, research has shown that there are a variety of solid benefits of olive oil consumption, including a decrease in the risk of breast cancer incidence in women.

3.   Dairy in moderation

While in some cases it can be helpful to eat low-Fat or non-Fat dairy products, many people worldwide rely on heavy creams, eggs, and other Fatty dairy products for their daily diets. The Mediterranean diet has low milk content. All dairy products which are currently on the menu are actually low in Fat. A person who consumes four eggs a week is considered an extremely heavy eater of the eggs.

4.   Red Meat in Moderation

Very little red meat is included in the Mediterranean diet. This diet depends on moderate amounts of lean poultry and fresh fish when it comes to meat products. As a result, people on the Mediterranean diet have lower levels of "bad" cholesterol and higher levels of "good: cholesterol". Furthermore, thanks to the inclusion of lean and fresh fish in the diet, the members of the Mediterranean diet enjoy the antioxidant benefits present in some oils and fish products.

5.   A Well Balanced Dieting Scheme

Ultimately, the Mediterranean diet is gaining worldwide acclaim from experts and adherents as it is a balanced diet program. Study after study shows that a balanced diet low in Fat which includes fruit, vegetables, whole grains and lean meatworks to ensure complete health and well-being.

Conclusion

The Mediterranean diet isn't only an approach to shied weight, however, it is an approach to completely transform you, and in doing as such, dragging out it. The medical advantages are perpetual, particularly when they are joined with work out, making this nourishment experience something unquestionably worth investigating. The primary concern is - the individuals who are on this eating regimen have lower death rates than the individuals who are not, which is reason enough to try it out. In the event that you have a past filled with coronary illness in your family, you truly can't stand to proceed in a similar way and now you have another option.

Healthy living is a treasured luxury that doesn't come by itself. You have to schedule it. Nutrition plays a crucial role in supplying the body with essential nutrients for growth and development. While some foods are considered healthy and in large quantities are required, others may be excluded from a daily diet. So works a Mediterranean diet plan.

The most common type of healthy diet is the Mediterranean diet. Studies have proved that people in the Mediterranean region can attribute the secret of healthy living to their balanced diet and active lifestyles. Researches have also shown that not only does this diet alleviate chronic heart disease, it also increases life expectancy.

Today's habits show that most people prefer to eat fried, frozen, or tinned foods that contain saturated

Fats and sugar. Lifestyles often suggest that most people don't take the time to exercise. As a result, with an increased chance of heart disease, diabetes and cancers, many people are obese and unhealthy.

The Mediterranean diet plan does not reduce the food types that one eats. The diet advises wise choices regarding food. For starters, instead of tinned and frozen food, one should eat fresh fruit and vegetables.

The food plan is based on the pyramid Mediterranean diet. According to him, cereals, grains, pasta, vegetables, legumes, beans, fruit, and nuts are food products to be included in a daily diet. These nutritious goods are a rich source of carbohydrates, fabrics, vitamins, minerals, and Proteins. The recommended milk, yogurt and cheese consumption, low to moderate, reduce excessive intake of saturated Fats. Animal meat such as chicken and eggs shall be consumed regularly and red meat, several times a month. Fish is considered a better choice, since it is high in nutritional value.

The combination of the products and principles mentioned above contribute to the success and strength of the Mediterranean diet, the perfect model of a balanced diet. If you eat a lot of vegetables but always cook them with butter, if you adopt wholemeal bread or if you often cook pulses but drink sodas throughout the day, the balance of the diet Mediterranean will not be there. This balance is achieved not over a day but a week (and over the long term!). You may well rush to a rib of beef and not eat meat for the next three days. Or enjoy a square of chocolate with your coffee.

Finally, remember that this Mediterranean diet is very satisfying thanks to the vegetables and wholemeal bread. If you have extra pounds, you will spontaneously eat less - especially if you take the time to chew well to activate your center of satiety - and you will lose them without a problem, without headache and frustration, above all. Also, you will be sure not to take them back because you will have integrated good eating habits. The good weather arrives with their procession of attractive vegetables: it's the right time to get started!

If you would still like to know more about this excellent diet, you can. You can find on the Internet a whole world of information on the Mediterranean diet, and many books have been written about it. At the end of the day, the Mediterranean diet is incredibly healthy and satisfying, and you will not be disappointed if you give it a try.

Printed in Great Britain
by Amazon